PreTest®
Step 3 Simulated Examination

PreTest®
Step 3 Simulated Examination

Editor

John R. Thornborough, Ph.D.

Mount Sinai School of Medicine
New York, New York

Contributors

Larry Binkovitz, M.D.
Katherine Teets Grimm, M.D.
H. Jay Wisnicki, M.D.

McGraw-Hill
Health Professions Division/PreTest® Series

New York St. Louis San Francisco Auckland
Bogotá Caracas Lisbon London Madrid
Mexico City Milan Montreal New Delhi
San Juan Singapore Sydney Tokyo Toronto

McGraw-Hill
A Division of The McGraw-Hill Companies

PreTest® Step 3 Stimulated Examination
International Editions 1997

1 2 3 4 5 6 7 8 9 0 SWN PMP 9 8 7 6

Figures for questions 27 and 297 from King, Geller, and Chabot, *Surgery: PreTest Self-Assessment and Review,* 7/e, New York: McGraw-Hill, 1995; with permission. Figures for questions 102 and 313 from Schaeffer, Bennet, and Kravath, *Pediatrics: PreTest Self-Assessment and Review,* 7/e, New York: McGraw-Hill, 1995; with permission. Figure for question 208 from Hovsepian, *Radiography: PreTest Self-Assessment and Review,* New York: McGraw-Hill, 1993; with permission. Figures for questions 64, 77, 212, 234, 258, 272, 284, 287 and 331 from Stone, *Harrison's Principles of Internal Medicine: PreTest Self-Assessment and Review,* 13/e, New York: McGraw-Hill, 1994; with permission. Figure for question 321 from Grossman, *Cardiac Catheterization and Angiography,* 3/e, Philadelphia: Lea & Febiger, 1986; with permission.

This book was set in Times Roman by ILOC, Inc.
The editors were Gail Gavert and Deborah L. Harvey.
The production supervisors were Anna Lieggi and Diana Porter Jones.

Library of Congress Cataloging-in-Publication Data
PreTest step 3 simulated examination / editor, John R. Thornborough.
p. cm.
Includes bibliographical references and index.
ISBN 0-07-052067-4
1. Medicine–Examinations, questions, etc. I. Thornborough, John R.
[DNLM: 1. Medicine–examination questions. W 18.2 P9425 1996]
R834.6.P743 1996
610'.76–dc20
DNLM/DLC 95-45520
for Library of Congress

When ordering this title, use ISBN 0-07-114610-5

Printed in Malaysia

Contents

Introduction

PreTest® Step 3 Simulated Examination has been designed to help physicians preparing for the United States Medical Licensing Examination (USMLE) Step 3.

The overall format of *PreTest® Step 3 Simulated Examination* – including the number, item type, and degree of difficulty of the questions, the use of illustrative materials, and the time limits imposed – is similar to the format of the actual Step 3 examination. However, because the USMLE examinations necessarily vary in both format and content from year to year, PreTest does not attempt to exactly duplicate the Step 3 examination; rather it presents standard multiple-choice questions on topics and problems, involving both basic concepts and recent advances that are of key importance in the clinical sciences.

The blueprint for *PreTest® Step 3 Simulated Examination* was designed to approximate that of the actual USMLE Step 3. As a consequence, *PreTest® Step 3 Simulated Examination* contains questions that may be categorized into one of three clinical encounter frames. Approximately 30 percent of the exam's questions concern the initial workup of the patient, 56 percent have to do with continued care, and 15 percent represent emergency situations. Overall, within these three encounter frames, 10 percent of the questions relate to the taking of a history and the performance of a physical examination, 13 percent to diagnostic studies, 15 percent to making a diagnosis, and 7 percent to offering a prognosis. Physician tasks involving the management of patients include health maintenance (10 percent), clinical intervention (17 percent), clinical therapeutics (15 percent), legal and ethical issues (1 percent), and the application of basic concepts (12 percent).

Approximately 25 percent of the questions in *PreTest® Step 3 Simulated Examination* are brand new and written specifically for this examination. The remainder of the questions are carefully selected and edited from the broad range of published PreTest material, with each item evaluated, reviewed, and updated for the Step 3 examination.

Each question is accompanied by the correct answer, a specific page reference to a current journal article, a comprehensive textbook, or both, and a brief explanation of the question.

PreTest's simulated Step 3 exam is approximately half the length of the actual Step 3 examination. It is divided into two sections of 200 questions each (the total number of questions equals 400), requiring one full day (7 hours) of testing. The USMLE Step 3 examination is divided into four sections of approximately 180 questions, each requiring two full days (approximately 12 hours) of testing.

Directions for Use

PREPARATION FOR THE EXAMINATION

In preparing for both the *PreTest® Step 3 Simulated Examination* and the actual exam, you will find it helpful to devise a plan for review that includes an analysis of your strengths and weaknesses, regular self-testing, and making and following a schedule of study. PreTest's *How to Prepare for the National Medical Board Examination Comprehensive Part I* can help you identify your strengths and weaknesses and design a plan of study whether you are preparing for USMLE Step 1, 2, or 3. Whatever you do, to ensure that you review efficiently and effectively and, therefore, do well on the Step 3 examination, your most important strategies are to plan a review program and schedule your time before the exam.

TYPES OF QUESTIONS

There are two basic types of questions in this examination:

Type 1 – One best-answer completion. A question or incomplete statement (often a patient description or clinical scenario) is followed by four or five answers or completions. You are to select the single best choice.

Type 2 – Matching questions. A group of 5 to 26 lettered answers or a lettered diagram is followed by a list of numbered phrases or statements. For each numbered phrase or statement, you are to select the one answer that is most closely related to it. Each answer may be selected once, more than once, or not at all.

Each type of question has only one best answer (unless otherwise indicated). Sometimes no clear-cut choice exists in a situation, as is the case in the actual practice of medicine. Therefore, although several choices may seem appealing, the less applicable ones must be rejected in favor of the single best answer. Make sure you do not mark more than one space per question unless instructed to do so.

TIME ALLOTMENT

The USMLE Step 3 examination allows approximately 65 seconds per question. In accordance with this time allotment, there is a $3^1/2$-hour limit for each of the two sections of *PreTest® Step 3 Simulated Examination*. Each section of this examination should be treated as a separate test. Thus, you should plan to take each section of this PreTest at a time when you will be undisturbed for a minimum of $3^1/2$ hours.

Choose a quiet, well-lit location, free from distractions. The area should be clear of books, papers, or other materials, and a clock or watch should be easily visible–ideally you should set an alarm clock to ring after $3^1/2$ hours. Have three sharpened No. 2 pencils and an eraser available. If a section is completed within the allotted time, any remaining time may be used to review questions in that section. Extra time from one section should **not** be spent in answering questions in another section.

INTERPRETING YOUR SCORES

After you have completed the examination (or individual section), you may score your examination using the answer key at the end of the book. In scoring, mark each incorrect answer with an "X" and subtract the number of questions with incorrect answers from the total number of questions in the examination (400) or individual section of the examination (200).

The **raw score** is the number of questions answered correctly.

The **percentage correct** is calculated by dividing the raw score by the number of items in the examination (400). On the actual USMLE Step 3 examination, a minimum passing score usually results from correctly answering 55 to 65 percent of the total number of questions in the test.

Percentile scores are also reported on the actual USMLE Step 3 examination. All examinees are first ranked according to their raw scores. Ranking is then expressed relative to the percentage of examinees who receive a lower score, that is, as a percentile score. For example, if you answer 223 questions correctly on this PreTest examination, you would have a raw score of 223, and a percentage correct of 56. If 66 percent of the people taking this examination answered fewer than 223 questions correctly, then your percentile score would be 66.

The USMLE uses a **standard score** system whereby the percentile score is then converted to a standard score. The mean score is set at 200 and one standard deviation equals 20. The minimum passing score of the actual Step 3 examination is a standard score of 176.

It is very important to realize that your PreTest scores may not accurately predict the scores you will attain on the USMLE Step 3 examination. Because your PreTest scores reflect your present level of knowledge, your standing relative to your colleagues may change between now and the time you take the official examination — especially if, in the interim, you study those areas in which your PreTest results indicate weakness.

WHEN YOU FINISH THE PreTest EXAMINATION

After answering the questions in either a section or the whole examination and calculating your score, spend as much time as you need verifying your answers and carefully reading the explanations. Although you should pay special attention to the explanations for the questions you answered incorrectly, you should read *every* explanation. The authors of this book have designed the explanations to reinforce and supplement the information tested by the questions. After you have read the explanation for a given question, if you feel you need still more information about material covered, consult the references indicated.

The answer key lists the correct answer, the Physician Task, and the Clinical Encounter Frame (Initial Workup, Continued Care, and Emergency Care). You may wish to calculate separate scores for each area to determine specifically where your strengths and weaknesses are located. Once you have done that, use most of your remaining review time for studying your weakest areas, since those are where you can make the most improvement and, thus, raise your total score. For more information on how to allocate your time among subjects as well as how to approach different question formats, see PreTest's *How to Prepare for the Step 1 Medical Exam,* 3/e.

Book A

Time: Three hours and thirty minutes

Number of items: 200

Book A

DIRECTIONS (Questions 1-116): Each question below contains four or five suggested responses. Select the **one best** response to each question.

1. A 42-year-old alcoholic with cirrhosis is hospitalized because of ascites and pitting edema. Laboratory values upon admission reveal:

Serum electrolytes (mmol/L): Na^+ 135; K^+ 3.1; Cl^- 98; HCO_3^- 27

Serum chemistries: BUN 5.4 mmol/L (15 mg/dL); creatinine 176 mmol/L (2.0 mg/dL)

Urine output is 400 ml/24 h with an osmolality of 640 mosmol/kg and sodium concentration of 7 mmol/L

Which of the following measures is likely to be most beneficial in the treatment of this patient's sodium retention?

(A) Abdominal paracentesis to drain 1.5 L of fluid daily

(B) Bed rest and a low-sodium diet

(C) Intravenous furosemide, 120 mg twice daily

(D) Intravenous mannitol, 25 g twice daily

(E) Oral furosemide, 120 mg twice daily

2. The earliest sign of female puberty is

(A) adrenarche

(B) menarche

(C) menopause

(D) onset of growth spurt

(E) thelarche

Questions 3-4: A 26-year-old man is brought to the emergency room following a 911 call. He apparently swallowed a handful of pills. The patient complains of shortness of breath and tinnitus, but refuses to identify the pills he ingested. Pertinent laboratory values are as follows:

Arterial blood gases:
pH 7.38; P_{O_2} 126 torr, P_{CO_2} 12 torr

Serum electrolytes (meq/L):
Na^+ 138; K^+ 4.8; Cl^- 102; HCO_3^- 8

3. How would you characterize this patient's acid-base disturbance?

(A) Acute respiratory alkalosis, compensated

(B) Chronic respiratory alkalosis, compensated

(C) Metabolic acidosis, compensated

(D) Mixed metabolic acidosis and respiratory acidosis

(E) Mixed metabolic acidosis and respiratory alkalosis

4. What is the most likely cause of the disturbance in this patient? An overdose of

(A) aspirin

(B) barbiturates

(C) diazepam (Valium)

(D) methanol

(E) phenformin

5. A 68-year-old hypertensive man underwent successful repair of a ruptured abdominal aortic aneurysm. He received 9 L Ringer's lactate solution and 4 units of whole blood during the operation. Two hours after transfer to the surgical intensive care unit, the following hemodynamic parameters are obtained:

Systemic blood pressure (BP): 90/60 mmHg

Pulse rate: 110 beats per minute

Central venous pressure (CVP): 7 mmHg

Pulmonary artery pressure: 28/10

Pulmonary capillary wedge pressure: 8 mmHg

Cardiac output: 1.9 L/min

Systemic vascular resistance: 35 Woods units (normal 24 to 30 Woods units)

Pa_{O_2}: 140 torr (FI_{O_2} 0.45)

Urine output: 15 mL/h (specific gravity 1.029)

Hematocrit: 35%

Proper management would now call for

(A) administration of a diuretic to increase urine output

(B) administration of a vasopressor agent to increase the systemic blood pressure

(C) administration of a fluid challenge to increase the urine output

(D) administration of a vasodilating agent to decrease the elevated systemic vascular resistance

(E) a period of observation to obtain more data

Questions 6-7: A 55-year-old man undergoes intravenous pyelography (IVP) as part of a workup for hypertension. A solitary radiolucent mass, 3 cm in size, is noted in the left kidney; the study otherwise is normal.

6. The man complains of no symptoms referable to the urinary tract, and examination of urine sediment is within normal limits. Which of the following studies should be performed next?

(A) CT scanning (with contrast enhancement) of the left kidney

(B) Early-morning urine collections for cytology (three samples)

(C) Renal ultrasonography

(D) Repeat intravenous pyelography in 6 months

(E) Selective renal arteriography

7. The renal mass is shown to be a simple cyst by sonography. The next appropriate step in the management of this mass is

(A) alcohol ablation of the renal cyst percutaneously

(B) cyst aspiration to insure the benign nature of the renal cyst

(C) repeat ultrasound in 6 months to insure stability

(D) screening of the patient's first degree relatives for renal cystic disease

(E) none of the above

8. Which of the following statements regarding acute glomerular nephritis is true?

(A) The presence of nephrosis is incompatible with the diagnosis of acute glomerular nephritis

(B) Hematuria usually is microscopic

(C) Leukocyte casts should suggest another renal lesion

(D) The presence of a crescentic glomerulonephritis on renal biopsy is a poor prognostic indicator

(E) The prognosis in children tends to be worse than the prognosis in adults

9. A 19-year-old woman sustains a deep laceration on the volar surface of the right wrist. Median nerve injury would result in

(A) a clawhand defect

(B) a sensory deficit only

(C) a wristdrop

(D) an inability to flex the metacarpophalangeal joints

(E) an inability to oppose the thumb to the other fingers

10. Achondroplasia, a congenital disorder of cartilage formation, is characterized by dwarfism. Which of the following statements about achondroplasia is true?

(A) The inheritance pattern is autosomal recessive

(B) Mutation accounts for 90 percent of all cases

(C) Cesarean section is rarely necessary

(D) Affected women rarely live to reproductive age

(E) All of the above

11. A patient presents with low serum sodium and chloride, normal potassium and bicarbonate, and a serum osmolality of 245 mosm/kg. Serum creatinine is normal. These findings suggest

(A) acute bacterial meningitis

(B) Addison's disease

(C) congestive heart failure

(D) diabetes mellitus

(E) multiple myeloma

12. Which of the following statements is true regarding renal cell carcinoma?

(A) Erythrocytosis is more common than anemia at presentation

(B) Development of a left scrotal varicocele indicates inoperability

(C) Patients with von Hippel-Lindau disease should be screened for renal cell carcinoma

(D) The presence of calcifications with a solid renal mass suggests a tumor other than renal cell carcinoma

(E) Lung metastases do not adversely affect prognosis

13. A 19-year-old male presents at the emergency room with a severe asthmatic attack. Initial treatment including bronchodilators is instituted. Which of the following will best document initial severity of the bronchoconstriction and response to therapy?

(A) Arterial blood gas measurement

(B) Chest radiography

(C) Measurement of peak expiratory flow or FEV_1

(D) Measurement of pulsus paradoxus

(E) Observation of accessory muscle use

Questions 14-15: During a bicycle accident, a 12-year-old girl sustains blunt abdominal trauma. She develops upper abdominal pain, nausea, and vomiting. She is brought to the emergency room.

14. An upper gastrointestinal series reveals a total obstruction of the duodenum with a "coiled spring" appearance in the second and third portions. This finding is likely due to

(A) duodenal hematoma

(B) duodenal laceration with contained perforation

(C) edematous ampulla of Vater

(D) intussusception

(E) pancreatic pseudocyst

15. Appropriate management of this patient is

(A) duodenal resection

(B) duodenojejunostomy

(C) gastrojejunostomy

(D) nasogastric suction and observation

(E) TPN to increase size of retropentoneal fat pad

16. A 27-year-old white woman has a maternal serum alpha-fetoprotein (MSAFP) at 18 weeks' gestation of 5.5 multiples of the median. What is the next most appropriate step in the workup of this markedly elevated maternal serum alpha-fetoprotein?

(A) A second MSAFP test

(B) Amniocentesis

(C) Amniography

(D) Recommendation of termination

(E) Ultrasound examination

17. A 40-year-old woman with new onset hemoptysis is found to have 2+ proteinuria and microscopic hematuria. BUN concentration is 7.1 mmol/L (20 mg/dL), and serum creatinine concentration is 177 μmol/L (2.0 mg/dL). Serologic findings include normal complement levels, increased immunoglobulin A levels, and a negative assay for fluorescent antinuclear antibodies. Renal biopsy reveals granulomatous necrotizing vasculitis with scattered immunoglobulin and complement deposits. The most likely diagnosis is

(A) Henoch-Schönlein purpura

(B) Goodpasture's syndrome

(C) mesangial lupus glomerulonephritis

(D) microscopic polyarteritis

(E) Wegener's granulomatosis

18. A young woman complains of chronic dyspnea and chest pain on exertion. Arterial blood-gases reveal a pH of 7.48, P_{O_2} 81 mmHg, and P_{CO_2} 32 mmHg. There is right axis deviation shown on EKG. Chest x-ray now shows enlarged pulmonary arteries but is otherwise normal, and a lung perfusion scan reveals mild inhomogeneity but no perfusion defects. Echocardiogram demonstrates right heart strain, but no primary cardiac disease. Which of the following is the most appropriate study to obtain in the diagnostic workup?

(A) Holter monitoring

(B) Open lung biopsy

(C) Right-heart catheterization

(D) Serum α_1-antitrypsin level

(E) Transbronchial biopsy

Questions 19-20: A 21-year-old college student with no prior medical problems begins working as a laboratory technician. He subsequently presents because of several recent episodes of shortness of breath, cough, fever, chills, and malaise. Each episode has lasted several days. The patient is seen during the recovery phase of such an episode; findings at physical examination are normal. Chest x-ray reveals several ill-defined, diffuse, patchy infiltrates. The laboratory evaluation is positive only for an increased erythrocyte sedimentation rate. Pulmonary function studies display reduced lung volumes.

19. On further questioning it is learned that these episodes begin on days the patient is required to tend to experiments involving laboratory rats at the animal facility. What is the best treatment for this condition?

(A) Discontinuation of visits to the animal facility

(B) Inhaled beclomethasone

(C) Inhaled cromolyn sodium

(D) Prednisone

(E) No treatment

20. The patient's chest x-ray later demonstrates hyperinflation of both lungs and tubular areas of opacity emanating from the upper hilar regions bilaterally suggesting allergic bronchopulmonary aspergillosis. Which of the following would support this diagnosis?

(A) Delayed, tuberculin-type skin-test reaction to *Aspergillus fumigatus*

(B) Marked elevation of serum immunoglobulin E level

(C) Presence of serum precipitins to *A. fumigatus*

(D) Radiographic evidence of bronchiectasis

(E) Sputum culture positive for *A. fumigatus*

---

21. A middle-aged man with a history of asthma presents to the emergency room with a nonproductive cough and dyspnea upon exertion. On examination you note a low-grade fever and a 10-kg (22-lb) weight loss over the past eight weeks. His white blood cell count is 13,500/mm^3. He is on no medications. A chest x-ray demonstrates peripheral pulmonary infiltrates. What is the most likely diagnosis?

(A) Alveolar proteinosis

(B) Chronic eosinophilic pneumonia

(C) Idiopathic pulmonary fibrosis

(D) Lymphangiomyomatosis

(E) Polymyositis

22. A 59-year-old woman presents whom you suspect has osteoporosis. Which of the following screening tools for osteoporosis is currently recommended for all menopausal women?

(A) Dual-photon absorptiometry

(B) Quantitative computed tomography

(C) Radiologic techniques are not appropriate

(D) Single-photon absorptiometry

(E) Spinal x-ray

Questions 23-24: A 19-year-old female develops adult respiratory distress syndrome after a complicated delivery. Breathing room air, she has the following arterial blood-gas values: pH 7.5, P_{O_2} 48 mmHg, and P_{CO_2} 28 mmHg. She shows only mildly improved oxygenation when breathing 80% oxygen by mask.

23. The predominant cause of hypoxemia in the woman described above would be

(A) a block in alveolar-capillary diffusion

(B) hypoventilation

(C) poor cardiac output

(D) right-to-left shunting

(E) ventilation-perfusion mismatch

24. The patient requires tracheal intubation and mechanical ventilation due to hypoxemia. Inspired oxygen concentration is 80%. Initially, she is agitated and fights the respirator. Arterial blood gases now show pH 7.20, P_{O_2} 75 mmHg, and P_{CO_2} 56 mmHg. The most appropriate management step at this time would be

(A) extubation

(B) to infuse sodium bicarbonate intravenously

(C) to initiate extracorporeal membrane oxygenation

(D) to raise the inspired oxygen concentration

(E) to sedate the woman and control her ventilation

25. Death rates from cancer have increased steadily over the past 40 years in primary cancers of the

(A) breast

(B) colon

(C) lung

(D) stomach

(E) uterus

26. Which of the following is the most frequent manifestation of neurologic abnormality in AIDS patients?

(A) Aseptic meningitis

(B) Myelopathy

(C) Peripheral neuropathy

(D) Primary CNS lymphoma

(E) Subacute encephalitis

27. The thyroid scan shown below exhibits a pattern that is most consistent with which of the following disorders?

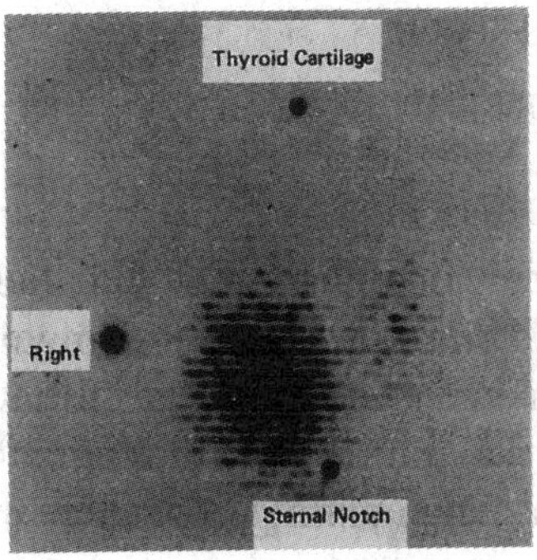

(A) Graves' disease

(B) Hypersecreting adenoma

(C) Lateral aberrant thyroid

(D) Medullary carcinoma of thyroid

(E) Papillary carcinoma of thyroid

28. Over the course of several months a middle-aged man has noted progressive weakness in his left leg. He also has had some trouble swallowing foods. There is marked atrophy with fasciculations in the muscles of both legs, hyperactive reflexes in the upper and lower extremities, a diminished gag reflex, and a positive extensor plantar response. Which of the following is the most likely diagnosis?

(A) Amyotrophic lateral sclerosis

(B) Cervical spondylosis

(C) Guillain-Barré syndrome

(D) Lambert-Eaton syndrome

(E) Vitamin-B_{12} deficiency

29. You are counseling a 47-year-old woman who has intraductal comedo carcinoma of the breast. What is the likelihood that she will sustain ipsilateral axillary lymph node metastases?

(A) Less than 5 percent

(B) 10 percent

(C) 20 percent

(D) 30 percent

(E) 40 percent

30. During an evaluation of renal function in a 23-year-old primigravida near term you observe an increased glomerular filtration rate. The renal glomerular filtration rate (GFR) can change during pregnancy by as much as

(A) -50 percent

(B) 0 percent

(C) 10 percent

(D) 50 percent

(E) 100 percent

31. A 35-year-old man comes to the emergency room at midnight because he has awakened from sleep three nights in a row with severe pain in and above his left eye. In addition he noted unusual tearing, nasal stuffiness, and a sense of swelling over his left cheek. Neurologic evaluation reveals left ptosis and miosis that disappear after the headache resolves. The most appropriate action is to

(A) obtain an emergency CT scan and, if results are normal, perform a lumbar puncture to search for evidence of subarachnoid hemorrhage

(B) reassure the patient that he has a characteristic clinical syndrome called cluster headache. It is benign and frequently responds to administration of ergotamine or lithium

(C) refer the patient to an ophthalmologist for evaluation of eye pain and pupillary change

(D) inform the patient that he has "classic migraine" and administer ergotamine, 1 mg four times a day

(E) evaluate diabetes mellitus in the patient

32. A 44-year-old man has had difficulty concentrating on his job recently. He has irregular, jerky movements of his extremities and fingers. An uncle, sister, and grandparent died in mental institutions and his mother became demented in middle age. The most likely diagnosis is

(A) alcoholic cerebral degeneration

(B) Gilles de la Tourette's disease

(C) Hallervorden-Spatz disease

(D) Huntington's chorea

(E) Wilson's disease

33. A 65-year-old woman with diabetes mellitus has a 3-month history of sacral pain. In the last month a burning pain progressively developed over the lateral aspect of her left foot and was followed by loss of sensation and weakness of plantar flexion and dorsiflexion. Electromyography showed fibrillations in the left gastrocnemius, extensor hallucis, and quadriceps muscles. Nerve conduction and a myelogram are normal. Now she complains that her knee "gives out" while walking; she has an absence of left knee and ankle jerks. Her physician should

(A) inform the patient that normal results on her myelogram make a diabetic neuropathy the most likely diagnosis

(B) arrange for a pelvic examination and schedule a CT scan of the pelvis to search for a malignancy compressing or infiltrating the lumbar-sacral plexus

(C) arrange for a repeat myelogram because of new quadriceps weakness

(D) arrange for a CT scan of the head to search for an expanding mass over the right sensorimotor strip that would affect the foot and leg

(E) reexamine her at 2-month intervals to determine progression of her condition

34. A 32-year-old woman complains of a bloody discharge from the nipple. Physical examination reveals a small, painful, movable nodule directly beneath the areola. The nipple itself is normal. The most likely diagnosis is

(A) cystosarcoma phylloides

(B) fibrocystic disease

(C) fibroadenoma

(D) intraductal papilloma

(E) medullary carcinoma

35. A 70-year-old man well known to you is brought in by his wife because of increased drowsiness and generally confused thinking over the past 2 months. Prior to a seemingly minor motor vehicle accident about 2 months ago, the patient had been running a small business without difficulty. A noncontrast CT scan of the brain is normal except that there are no cortical sulci and the ventricles are small. There are no focal or lateralizing signs on neurologic examination. The most likely diagnosis is

(A) Alzheimer's disease

(B) cerebrovascular accident

(C) depression

(D) metabolic encephalopathy

(E) subdural hematoma

36. A 26-year-old female patient has one child with a neural tube defect and is now pregnant again. Which of the following statements concerning neural tube defects is true?

(A) The overall incidence in the United States is 2 to 3 percent

(B) Levels of alpha-fetoprotein in maternal serum are constant throughout the gestational period

(C) Increased levels of alpha-fetoprotein in amniotic fluid are well correlated with severity of the lesion present

(D) Amniocentesis and detailed ultrasound evaluation of the fetus can accurately diagnose 95 to 99 percent of all cases of neural tube defects

(E) There is little recurrent risk of neural tube defects

37. During an otherwise normal examination of a noncyanotic 2-day-old baby, a systolic murmur associated along the left sternal border is detected. What is the most likely cause of the murmur?

(A) Patent ductus arteriosus
(B) Tetralogy of Fallot
(C) Transposition of the great vessels
(D) Tricuspid atresia
(E) Ventricular septal defect

38. In a comatose patient, cold-water irrigation of the right external auditory canal leads to deviation of both eyes to the right for 2 min followed by a slow drift back to the midline. This finding is most consistent with a lesion in the

(A) cerebral hemispheres
(B) pons
(C) right cerebellum
(D) right cochlea
(E) right labyrinth

39. A 64-year-old woman presents with a headache of one week duration thought to be due to stress. For the last 6 weeks she has had an increase in the severity of the headache and difficulty reading. Her husband has noted a mild but progressive intellectual decline in his wife during this period. On examination, she has grasping reactions and myoclonic jerks when loud noises occur. CT scan and cerebrospinal fluid examination are normal. The most likely diagnosis is

(A) Alzheimer's disease
(B) bilateral subdural hematoma
(C) Creutzfeldt-Jakob disease
(D) multiple sclerosis
(E) subacute sclerosing panencephalitis

Questions 40-41: A 32-year-old female patient is referred to a neurology clinic for the provisional diagnosis of multiple sclerosis.

40. The most common presenting finding or symptom to be expected is

(A) cerebellar ataxia
(B) internuclear ophthalmoplegia
(C) optic neuritis
(D) transverse myelitis
(E) urinary retention

41. Examination confirms the referral diagnosis. Which of the following is a true statement regarding multiple sclerosis?

(A) Magnetic resonance imaging will show abnormalities in greater than 90 percent of patients with multiple sclerosis
(B) Visual blurring may be due to optic neuritis or internuclear ophthalmoplegia
(C) Early adult onset tends to have a more favorable prognosis than late adult onset
(D) Seizures, fasiculations, and peripheral neuropathies are sufficiently rare as to call into question the diagnosis of multiple sclerosis
(E) All of the above are true

42. A 3-year-old child with congenital cyanosis most probably is suffering from

(A) patent ductus arteriosus
(B) tetralogy of Fallot
(C) transposition of the great vessels
(D) tricuspid atresia
(E) ventricular septal defect

43. A 55-year-old woman presents because of intermittent, brief, extreme stabbing pains in her lips and right cheek. The pain can be brought on by touching her face. The results of examination of the structures of the face and cranial nerves are entirely normal. Appropriate initial treatment for this condition would be

(A) amitriptyline

(B) carbamazepine

(C) ergotamine

(D) propranolol

(E) referral to an otolaryngologist for nerve block

44. A 21-year-old patient comes into the emergency department complaining of lower abdominal pain. Her β-hCG level is 5400 mIU/ml. The most appropriate diagnostic test at this time would be

(A) culdocentesis

(B) determination of serum progesterone

(C) laparoscopy

(D) transabdominal sonography

(E) transvaginal sonography

45. While wrestling with his young son, a 32-year-old man suddenly develops a severe headache, then lapses into unconsciousness. Examination in the emergency room reveals retinal hemorrhages, nuchal rigidity, and nominal eye movements on passive head rotation. The best initial diagnostic measure would be

(A) bilateral carotid and vertebral angiography

(B) CT scan of the head

(C) lumbar puncture

(D) radionuclide brain scan

(E) skull x-rays

46. The emergency room staff is confronted with a comatose patient with a severe head injury. The physician should

(A) perform a skull and neurologic examination, obtain a CT scan of the head, and recommend burr holes if the pupils are enlarged

(B) stabilize the neck, administer mannitol and steroids, and obtain a CT scan

(C) treat hypotension, ensure airway patency, perform a skull and neurologic examination, and obtain a CT scan

(D) treat hypoxia and hypotension, raise the head, and obtain a CT scan

(E) stabilize the neck, obtain neck and skull x-rays, and recommend burr holes if the pupils are enlarged

47. A 56-year-old woman well known to you because of a history of hypertension and diabetes has had profuse, watery diarrhea for 3 months. Laboratory studies of fecal water show the following:

Sodium: 39 mmol/L

Potassium: 96 mmol/L

Chloride: 15 mmol/L

Bicarbonate: 40 mmol/L

Osmolality: 270 mosmol/kgH_2O (serum osmolality: 280 mosmol/kgH_2O)

The most likely diagnosis is

(A) lactose intolerance

(B) laxative abuse

(C) nontropical sprue

(D) pancreatic insufficiency

(E) villous adenoma

48. A man brought into an emergency room is unresponsive and is displaying posturing. Pupils are 4 mm in size and react to light. No eye movements occur with head turning (oculocephalic maneuver) or with ice-water irrigation of the ear canals. The most likely diagnosis is

(A) bilateral internal carotid artery occlusion

(B) brain death

(C) brainstem hemorrhage

(D) drug ingestion

(E) hysteria-conversion coma

49. Following evacuation of a hydatiform molar pregnancy found at 12 weeks gestation in a patient who has no clinical or imaging findings of metastatic disease, appropriate follow-up would consist of

(A) combination chemotherapy

(B) hysterectomy

(C) radiation therapy

(D) single-agent chemotherapy

(E) weekly hCG titers

50. A 25-year-old man is brought to the emergency room with an excruciating headache of sudden onset. He has not suffered loss of consciousness. Physical examination does not disclose any evidence of focal neurologic deficit. The most likely diagnosis is

(A) carotid artery occlusion

(B) epidural hematoma

(C) meningioma

(D) ruptured berry aneurysm

(E) subdural hematoma

51. A 54-year-old man with peptic ulcer disease has been using aluminum hydroxide-containing antacids for the past several years to treat his symptoms. He complains of diffuse bone pain and progressive muscular weakness. These symptoms are most likely a result of

(A) aluminum intoxication

(B) aluminum-induced osteomalacia

(C) chronic phosphorus depletion

(D) malnutrition associated with his ulcer symptoms

(E) occult gastric malignancy

52. A simple drainage did not cure a patient's vesicovaginal fistula and you are about to surgically correct the problem. What is the most common cause of vesicovaginal fistulae in the United States?

(A) Abdominal hysterectomy

(B) Obstetric injury

(C) Radiation treatment

(D) Radical hysterectomy for cervical cancer

(E) Vaginal hysterectomy

53. A 36-year-old woman has noticed the absence of menses for the last 4 months. A pregnancy test is negative. Serum levels of luteinizing hormone and follicle-stimulating hormone are elevated, and the serum estradiol level is low. These findings suggest

(A) bilateral tubal obstruction

(B) exogenous estrogen administration

(C) panhypopituitarism

(D) polycystic ovarian disease

(E) premature menopause

Questions 54-55: A 42-year-old, obese man is admitted to the hospital for severe right-upper-quadrant pain suggestive of cholecystitis. During the first 2 days of hospitalization he is afebrile and has normal white blood cell counts, liver function tests, and oral cholecystogram. On the third day clusters of small vesicles are noted on the right upper abdomen extending laterally around to the right side of his back. His right-upper-quadrant pain became more intense.

54. A helpful diagnostic test to determine the cause of his pain would be

(A) endoscopic retrograde cholangiopancreatography (ERCP)

(B) exploratory laparotomy

(C) Giemsa stain of cellular material from the base of a vesicle

(D) percutaneous liver biopsy

(E) right-upper-quadrant ultrasound

55. Appropriate therapy for his condition would include

(A) cholecystectomy

(B) intravenous antibiotic therapy

(C) topical acyclovir

(D) topical fluorinated steroids

(E) none of the above

---

56. A 34-year-old woman has had three hospital admissions during the last year because of nephrolithiasis. The rate of 24-h urinary calcium excretion has been above the normal range on all three occasions and serum calcium concentrations were between 2.5 and 2.8 mmol/L (10.2 and 11.5 mg/dL). The serum phosphorus concentration was 0.77 mmol/L (2.4 mg/dL) and the parathyroid hormone level was 229 nL eq/mL (normal less than 150 nL eq/mL). The most appropriate management at this time would be

(A) to begin administration of prednisone, 40 mg daily, and taper the dose over a period of 4 weeks

(B) to administer thiazide diuretics to decrease calcium excretion

(C) symptomatic treatment of renal lithiasis only

(D) calcium supplementation to prevent progressive bone loss

(E) surgical exploration of the neck

57. Which of the following would not be expected in a patient with hypercalcemia due to sarcoidosis?

(A) An abnormal chest x-ray

(B) Hypercalciuria

(C) Hypergammaglobulinemia

(D) Increased absorption of calcium from the gastrointestinal tract

(E) Increased serum parathyroid hormone level

58. Upon examination, a 63-year-old woman is given a preliminary diagnosis of endometrial carcinoma. What is the hallmark symptom of this disease?

(A) Bloating

(B) Hemoptysis

(C) Postmenopausal bleeding

(D) Vaginal discharge

(E) Weight loss

59. A 21-year-old woman is examined because of secondary amenorrhea. Cyclic menses had commenced at the age of 14 years. When she was 19 years old she became pregnant and was hospitalized during the sixth month of that pregnancy because of bleeding and hypotension that proved to be the result of a spontaneous abortion with retained placental fragments; she received ten units of blood, and a dilation and curettage was performed. No menses have occurred during the 2 years since the hospitalization. She now wishes to become pregnant. Findings on physical examination, including rectopelvic examination, are normal. Results on complete blood counts, SMA-12, and chest x-ray are within normal limits. Serum thyroxine (T_4) concentration is 90 nmol/L (7 µg/dL) and an 8 A.M. plasma cortisol measurement is 470 nmol/L (17 µg/dL). No menstrual bleeding occurs after administration of 10 mg medroxyprogesterone acetate per day for 10 days or cyclic estrogen and progestogen (1.25 mg conjugated estrogens by mouth each day for 3 weeks with 10 mg medroxyprogesterone acetate per day for the last 7 days). At this point the most appropriate diagnostic study would be

(A) chromosomal analysis

(B) CT scan of the pituitary with contrast

(C) CT scan of the abdomen followed by wedge resection of the ovaries

(D) hysterosalpingogram

(E) metyrapone test

60. Acute renal failure is characterized by which of the following?

(A) Azotemia

(B) Irreversibility

(C) Oliguria

(D) Renal pathology

(E) Uremic syndrome

61. Which of the following statements concerning nasopharyngeal cancer is true?

(A) It has an unusually high incidence among Chinese

(B) It occurs primarily after the sixth decade of life

(C) It undergoes early metastasis to the lungs

(D) The treatment of choice is wide surgical excision of the primary tumor

(E) Initial evaluation should involve a biopsy of the primary tumor and neck nodes

62. Which of the following statements concerning Zenker's diverticulum is true?

(A) Aspiration pneumonitis is relatively rare

(B) It is an inherited abnormality

(C) The most common symptom is painful swallowing

(D) It is located at the pharyngoesophageal junction

(E) Surgical treatment is rarely required

63. A 48-year-old obese male with known gastroesophageal reflux presents to your office after three episodes of dysphagia while eating steak and chicken such that he could not swallow but rather had to vomit out the food. Which of the following should be further evaluated as likely causes given his symptoms?

(A) Achalasia

(B) Barrett's stricture

(C) Esophageal adenocarcinoma

(D) Peptic stricture

(E) All of the above

64. A 38-year-old woman is hospitalized for an upper gastrointestinal hemorrhage. Following an uneventful recovery, an upper gastrointestinal series (part of which is reproduced below) is obtained.

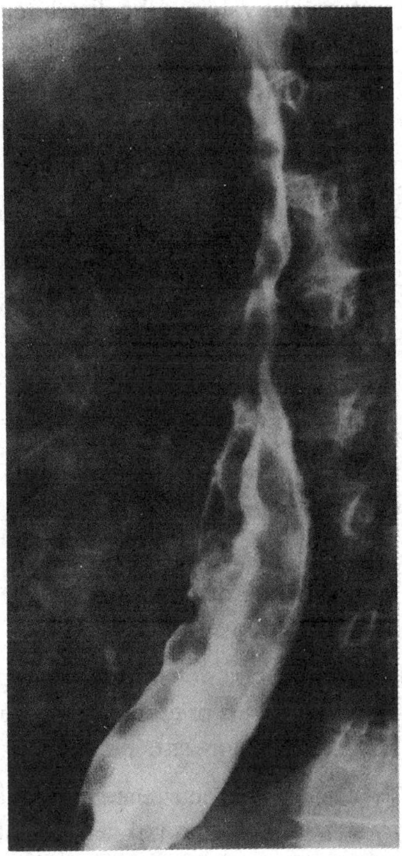

The abnormality demonstrated in the x-ray suggests which of the following diagnoses?

(A) Erosive gastritis

(B) Gastric ulcer

(C) Hiatal hernia

(D) Laënnec's cirrhosis

(E) Reflux esophagitis

65. True statements concerning AIDS and pregnancy include which of the following?

(A) The rate of perinatal transmission of human immunodeficiency virus (HIV) from infected pregnant women is unknown, but is probably low

(B) There is no need to delay the onset of pregnancy in women who are HIV antibody-positive, but show no manifestation of the disease

(C) Cesarean section delivery has been shown to be of benefit in preventing perinatal transmission of HIV

(D) Infected women should be advised against breastfeeding to avoid postnatal transmission

66. A 28-year-old nurse has been found to have chronic hepatitis C upon routine screening prior to a blood transfusion. Which of the following statements is true?

(A) Progression to cirrhosis occurs in at least 80 percent of patients with chronic hepatitis C

(B) Liver biopsy is usually normal in asymptomatic individuals

(C) Glucocorticoids should be used whenever the transaminase levels increase to twice greater than the baseline

(D) Loss of detectable hepatitis C virus (HCV) RNA during interferon therapy does not preclude relapse

(E) Reinfection of HCV following liver transplant is not common but if it occurs will usually lead to allograft failure

67. Four months ago, a 36-year-old man with a peptic ulcer underwent a Billroth II anastomosis, antrectomy, vagotomy, and gastrojejunostomy. He now returns for evaluation of an anastomotic ulcer. Fasting serum gastrin level is 350 ng/L; 5 min after intravenous infusion of secretin the serum gastrin level is 100 ng/L. The man should be advised that the most appropriate treatment for his condition is

(A) total vagotomy

(B) total gastrectomy

(C) resection of the distal antrum attached to the duodenal stump

(D) laparotomy to search for a gastrin-producing tumor

(E) medical therapy with liquid antacids

68. Which of the following statements regarding spermicides such as vaginal foams, creams, and suppositories is true?

(A) These agents often contain nonoxynol 9

(B) Effectiveness is independent of the concomitant use of condoms

(C) Effectiveness is higher in younger users

(D) Effectiveness is greater than that of the diaphragm

(E) These agents are associated with an increased incidence of congenital malformations

69. Which of the following is true regarding Meckel's diverticulum (MD)?

(A) Premalignant potential is increased with the size of diverticulum

(B) Usually found within 100 cm of the ileocecal valve in the distal ileum or colon

(C) A technetium-labeled RBC scan is most helpful in detecting symptomatic Meckel's diverticulum

(D) Usually not a cause of a leadpoint for intussusception

(E) Remnant of the omphalomesenteric duct

70. A patient is recently diagnosed with adenocarcinoma of the colon. Which of the following statements is true?

(A) The likelihood of developing a second colon carcinoma is not increased over baseline

(B) Elevated carcinoembryonic antigen (CEA) levels preoperatively are a positive prognostic indicator

(C) Anastomotic recurrence is frequent even when the initial margins of resection are tumor-free

(D) The presence of regional lymph node metastases will decrease the 5-year survival to 30 to 60 percent

(E) Carcinoma limited to the mucosa and submucosa is staged as Dukes C

71. It is important to identify and treat occult or early sepsis before it progresses to septic shock and the associated complications of multiple organ failure. Which of the following signs and symptoms may be expected in a patient with early sepsis?

(A) Hypoglycemia

(B) Increased arteriovenous oxygen difference

(C) Ongoing requirement of fluid resuscitation

(D) Metabolic acidosis

(E) Intermittent hypertension

72. Lactated Ringer's solution is being administered to a patient to replace gastrointestinal losses and to correct extracellular fluid deficit. Which of the following statements regarding lactated Ringer's solution is true?

(A) It contains the same concentration of sodium ions as does plasma

(B) It can be given in large quantities without seriously affecting acid-base balance

(C) It has a pH of approximately 7.0

(D) It is isosmotic with plasma

(E) All of the above

73. A 52-year-old woman is hospitalized for medical management of severe alcoholic hepatitis. On the ninth hospital day she develops a temperature of 38.3°C (101°F) and generalized abdominal discomfort. Abdominal examination reveals significant and diffuse abdominal tenderness without guarding; hepatosplenomegaly is present but is unchanged from the admission examination. Rectal and pelvic examinations reveal no area of localized tenderness; stool guaiac testing is positive. Hematocrit is 27 percent, white blood cell count is 12,000/mm^3, and liver function tests are unchanged from admission—total serum bilirubin, 214 µmol/L (12.5 mg/dL); serum AST, 2.5 µkat/L (150 Karmen units/mL); and serum alkaline phosphatase, 180 units. The procedure most likely to yield diagnosis information in this case would be

(A) abdominal sonography

(B) blood culture

(C) paracentesis

(D) serum amylase determination

(E) supine and upright x-rays of the abdomen

74. Which of the following statements is true regarding acute pancreatitis?

(A) The majority of cases are self-limited and without long-term sequelae

(B) The presence of pancreatic necrosis and peripancreatic inflammation and fluid collections on CT scans (severity score greater than 7) indicate a mortality of 15 to 20 percent

(C) Ten percent of patients will go on to develop a pancreatic abscess

(D) Urgent ERCP should be undertaken in patients with presumed gallstone pancreatitis and the presence of three or more Ranson factors

(E) All of the above

75. Which of the following statements concerning appendicitis during pregnancy is true?

(A) Diagnosis is relatively straightforward

(B) The maternal death rate increases as gestational age increases

(C) Surgical treatment should be delayed until the diagnosis is firmly established

(D) The incidence is generally lowered by pregnancy

(E) The rate of fetal loss is less than 5 percent

76. What is the most common etiology of mechanical obstruction of the colon?

(A) Adhesions

(B) Carcinoma

(C) Hernia

(D) Sigmoid diverticulitis

(E) Volvulus

77. A 28-year-old man has had diarrhea and crampy right lower quadrant abdominal pain for the last 4 weeks. During the last 10 days, he also has had episodic low-grade fever, abdominal distention, and anorexia without vomiting but leading to a weight loss of 3.2 kg (7 lb). On examination, he is mildly uncomfortable. Vital signs are temperature, 37.8°C (100.1°F); pulse, 100 beats per minute; and blood pressure, 110/60 mmHg. His sclerae are anicteric, and there is no palpable lymphadenopathy. A tender, indistinct fullness is palpable in the right lower quadrant of the abdomen, but otherwise the abdomen is soft and without rebound tenderness or palpable hepatosplenomegaly. Rectal examination reveals no masses or focal tenderness, but the stool is guaiac-positive. Laboratory values include a hematocrit of 30 percent and a white blood cell count of 11,300/mm^3 with a shift to the left. Flat-plate and upright x-rays of the abdomen show some air-filled loops of small bowel but no air-fluid levels. Sigmoidoscopy is unremarkable. On barium enema examination, barium fails to reflux into the terminal ileum, but the colon is otherwise normal. A representative film from a small-bowel barium examination is shown below.

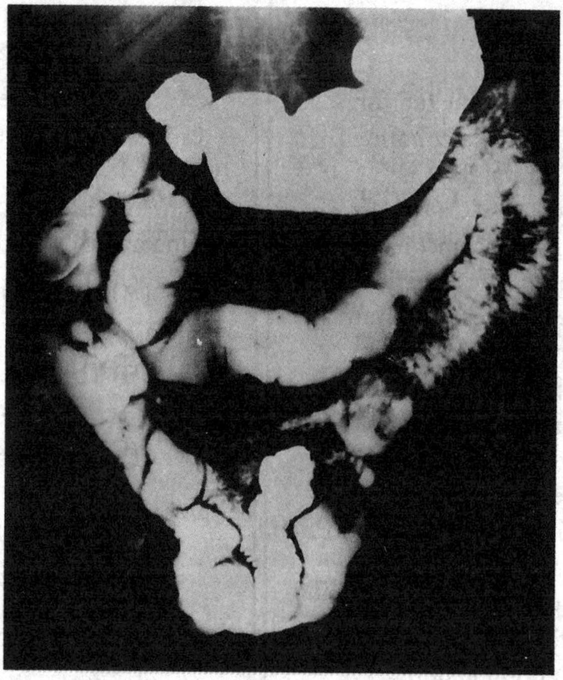

Which of the following disorders is most consistent with the clinical picture described?

(A) Adenocarcinoma of the small intestine

(B) Lymphoma of the small intestine

(C) Perforated appendix with appendiceal abscess

(D) Regional enteritis

(E) Whipple's disease

78. Four days after completing a 10-day course of ampicillin for urinary tract infection, a 39-year-old female develops bloody diarrhea, fever, and abdominal pain. Sigmoidoscopy demonstrates a hyperemic mucosa studded with plaquelike lesions. The most likely diagnosis is

(A) amebic colitis

(B) ischemic colitis

(C) pseudomembranous colitis

(D) *Shigella* superinfection

(E) toxic megacolon

79. The risk of having a baby with Down syndrome for a 30-year-old woman increases

(A) if the father of the baby is age 38

(B) if her pregnancy has been achieved by menotropin-induced ovulation

(C) if she had a previous baby with Turner syndrome (45,X)

(D) if she has had multiple first-trimester spontaneous abortions

(E) all of the above

80. Which of the following characteristics is more apt to be associated with Hodgkin's disease than with non-Hodgkin's lymphoma?

(A) "B" syndrome

(B) Extralymphatic presentation

(C) Dissemination at the time of diagnosis

(D) Involvement of Waldeyer's ring

(E) Most common type (60 percent) of lymphoma

81. Which of the following statements describes the relationship between testicular tumors and serum markers?

(A) Pure seminomas produce α-feto-protein (AFP) or β-human chorionic gonadotropin (β-hCG) in more than 90 percent of cases

(B) More than 40 percent of nonseminomatous germ cell tumors produce no cell markers

(C) Both β-hCG and AFP should be measured in following the progress of a tumor

(D) Measurement of tumor markers the day following surgery for localized disease is useful in determining completeness of the resection

(E) β-hCG is limited in its usefulness as a marker because it is identical to human luteinizing hormone

82. Of the following neoplasms, which is of a non-B-lymphocyte lineage?

(A) Burkitt's lymphoma

(B) Chronic lymphocytic leukemia

(C) Follicular lymphomas

(D) Mycosis fungoides

(E) Small lymphocytic (well-differentiated) lymphomas

83. A bicornuate uterus is associated with

(A) failure of complete fusion of the müllerian duct system

(B) a decrease in obstetric complications

(C) a decrease in urinary tract anomalies

(D) ovarian agenesis

84. Regarding constrictive pericarditis, which of the following statements is true?

(A) The hemodynamic pressure curve, the so-called square root sign, helps to distinguish this disorder from a restrictive cardiomyopathy

(B) Kussmaul's sign is negative

(C) The hemodynamic abnormality is due to impeded ventricular filling in late diastole

(D) Right and left atrial pressures are equalized and usually lowered

(E) Pericardial calcification and thickening cannot reliably be demonstrated with CT scanning due to cardiac motion

85. A 42-year-old woman has bilateral ankle edema of recent onset. On examination, her jugular venous pulse is 5 cmH_2O and the hepatojugular reflux is negative. The physical findings rule out which of the following possible causes of the pedal edema?

(A) Cyclic edema

(B) Hypoalbuminemia

(C) Pelvic thrombophlebitis

(D) Right heart failure

(E) Venous varicosities

86. Determination of central venous pressure is an integral part of the overall hemodynamic assessment of a patient. This pressure may be elevated by which of the following factors?

(A) Decreased venous tone

(B) Hypovolemia

(C) Increased depth of inspiration

(D) Pneumothorax

(E) Vasodilator drugs

87. Following surgery on an obese 52-year-old male, which of the following prophylactic regimens should be undertaken to help prevent post-operative pulmonary thromboembolism?

(A) Early ambulation

(B) Elastic stockings

(C) Dipyridamole (Persantine)

(D) Low-dose heparin

(E) None required, patient is not at serious risk

88. Which of the following statements regarding right ventricular infarctions is true?

(A) They frequently occur in isolation

(B) Volume expansion is contraindicated if there is elevated central venous pressure

(C) The hemodynamic alterations are similar to constrictive pericarditis

(D) The hypotension associated with RV infarctions is usually due to hormonal-related mechanisms

89. Regarding thrombolytic therapy in the treatment of acute myocardial infarction, which of the following statements is true?

(A) If treatment begins within 24 h of the onset of chest discomfort, it is likely that benefit will occur

(B) In comparison with streptokinase, tissue plasminogen activator (tPA) reduces mortality

(C) Reelevation of ST segments 24 h after the administration of streptokinase indicates reperfusion

(D) Aspirin and heparin should be administered after thrombolytic therapy

(E) None of the above

90. A 19-year-old male complains of a 7-day history of fever and chest pain. He was recently discharged from the hospital following treatment for injuries from a motor vehicle accident. Your examination demonstrates a leatherly to-and-fro friction rub at the lower left sternal border. Laboratory abnormalities include leukocytosis and an elevated sedimentation rate. Which of the following statements is true?

(A) The patient is unlikely to have another episode from this illness

(B) The symptoms are typically self-limited

(C) Cardiac tamponade is a frequent complication and prophylactic pericardiectomy should be performed

(D) Generally, glucocorticoids are required to alleviate chest pain and fever

(E) Aspirin is contraindicated because of the high incidence of hypersensitivity reaction associated with this illness

91. A 37-year-old woman with a 6-month history of "hives" and joint soreness comes to the local health clinic. Sedimentation rate obtained now is 85 mm/h. The procedure most likely to yield the correct diagnosis in this case would be

(A) a battery of wheal-and-flare allergy skin tests

(B) measurement of C1 esterase inhibitor activity

(C) measurement of total serum immunoglobulin E (IgE) concentration

(D) patch testing

(E) skin biopsy

92. A 47-year-old man has had fever, weight loss, arthralgias, pleuritic chest pain, and midabdominal pain for the last 2 months. One week ago he noticed difficulty dorsiflexing his right great toe. Blood pressure is 150/95 mmHg (he has always been normotensive), and laboratory studies reveal anemia of chronic disease, high erythrocyte sedimentation rate, and polymorphonuclear leukocytosis. The most likely diagnosis is

(A) allergic granulomatosis

(B) giant cell arteritis

(C) hypersensitivity vasculitis

(D) polyarteritis nodosa

(E) Wegener's granulomatosis

93. A 62-year-old white male has been seen in your office for two episodes of pneumonia in the past 3 months. He now presents with right flank pain and fever. Upon questioning he admits to nagging back and rib cage pain for several weeks. He is found to be anemic and has proteinuria. If the patient has myeloma, which of the following statements is true?

(A) An M protein in the urine would be a rare finding and suggests light chain disease

(B) Renal failure will occur within 2 years of diagnosis

(C) IgG paraproteinemia is associated with hyperviscosity more frequently than IgM or IgA paraproteinemia

(D) Benign monoclonal gammopathy could be excluded if the labeling index was less than 1 percent

(E) Splenomegaly and lymphadenopathy are common findings in typical myeloma

94. A 19-year-old woman with adrenocortical insufficiency is diagnosed with Addison's disease. Signs and symptoms of Addison's disease include

(A) hyperglycemia

(B) hypertension

(C) hypokalemia

(D) hyponatremia

(E) hypothermia

95. The hyperviscosity syndrome is most characteristic of which of the following plasma cell disorders?

(A) Heavy chain disease

(B) Indolent myeloma

(C) Multiple myeloma

(D) Primary amyloidosis

(E) Waldenström's macroglobulinemia

96. Which of the following conditions is associated with pubertal delay?

(A) Androgen excess

(B) Anorexia nervosa

(C) Chronic disease

(D) Gonadal dysgenesis

(E) All of the above

97. As a description of a woman's obstetric history, the digits 7-2-1-6 indicate that she has

(A) given birth to six term infants

(B) had two premature deliveries

(C) been pregnant seven times

(D) had two abortions

98. Characteristics of the blind loop syndrome include which of the following?

(A) Bacterial overgrowth is present in the small intestine

(B) Intestinal obstruction usually is present

(C) It is accompanied by microcytic anemia

(D) It nearly always requires surgical correction

(E) It is most common in neonates

99. In which of the following clinical situations would a diagnosis of ankylosing spondylitis most likely be correct?

(A) For the last 10 years, a 28-year-old man has had low back pain and stiffness, worse at night and relieved with activity

(B) For the last 5 years, a 32-year-old man has had low back pain made worse with activity but improved with bed rest

(C) For the last 10 years, a 34-year-old man has had intermittent bouts of mild low back pain; now, however, he suddenly is unable to dorsiflex his right great toe

(D) For the last 10 years, a 65-year-old man has had low back pain radiating down both posterior thighs to the knees

(E) For the last 15 years, a 72-year-old man has had progressive low back pain made worse with walking but improved with rest and leaning forward

100. Which of the following statements regarding rape, incest, and abuse is true?

(A) Most rape victims are attractive women between 20 and 30 years of age

(B) The chance of pregnancy occurring as a result of a rape episode is small

(C) Incestual activity is very uncommon

(D) Most cases of the sexual abuse of a child involve childcare workers

101. Which of the following statements concerning Meckel's diverticulum is correct?

(A) It is located on the mesenteric border of the ileum

(B) It is approximately 6 to 10 feet from the ileocecal valve

(C) Bleeding is the most common complication in affected adults

(D) Diverticula may contain gastric mucosa

102. An infant who has achromic skin patches (pictured) develops infantile spasms.

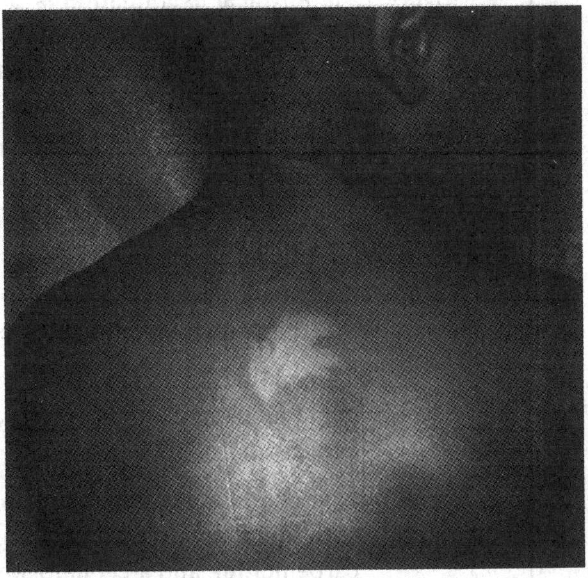

The disorder most likely to be affecting this infant is

(A) incontinentia pigmenti

(B) neurofibromatosis

(C) pityriasis rosea

(D) psoriasis

(E) tuberous sclerosis

103. Which of the following statements regarding the renal involvement associated with systemic lupus erythematosus is true?

(A) Clinically apparent renal disease occurs in 90 percent of affected persons

(B) Interstitial nephritis is a rare finding on renal biopsy

(C) Renal biopsy is not initially necessary in patients with deteriorating renal function and active urine sediment

(D) Renal disease is uncommon in patients with high-titer anti-double-stranded DNA antibodies

(E) Urinalysis in affected persons usually reveals proteinuria but little sediment and no red blood cells

104. A 22-year-old male presents with oral ulcerations and has a history of similar genital lesions on two occasions. Which of the following statements is true regarding Behçet's syndrome?

(A) It is best considered an autoimmune vasculitis

(B) Ulcerations may be chronic and heal with extensive fibrosis

(C) In this patient, the presence of iritis and posterior uveitis would argue against a diagnosis of Behçet's syndrome

(D) Peripheral vein thrombosis occurs in over 75 percent of patients

(E) Long-term disability and increased mortality necessitate aggressive treatment in this disorder

105. Dysmenorrhea

(A) is classified as primary if it is not related to detectable pelvic pathology

(B) incapacitates, if untreated, the majority of menstruating women

(C) usually occurs in anovulatory cycles

(D) is caused by psychologic factors in a major proportion of cases

(E) all of the above

106. A 28-year-old man with newly diagnosed acute myelogenous leukemia spikes a temperature to 38.7°C (101.7°F) on the sixth day of induction therapy. He feels well and has no physical complaints. His only medicine is intravenous cytosine arabinoside, 140 mg every 12 h. Physical examination is unrevealing. His white blood count is 900/mm^3, of which 10 percent are granulocytes and the rest mostly lymphocytes; platelet count is 24,000/mm^3. Findings on chest x-ray and urinalysis are normal. After obtaining appropriate cultures, the man's physician should

(A) observe closely for the development of a clinically evident source of fever

(B) begin antibiotic therapy with gentamicin, carbenicillin, and a cephalosporin

(C) begin granulocyte transfusion and antibiotic therapy with gentamicin, carbenicillin, and a cephalosporin

(D) begin gammaglobulin treatment and antibiotic therapy with gentamicin, carbenicillin, and a cephalosporin

(E) begin antibiotic therapy with amphotericin, gentamicin, carbenicillin, and a cephalosporin

107. A 50-year-old woman has had Raynaud's phenomenon of the hands for 15 years. The condition has become worse during the last year, and she has developed arthralgias and arthritis involving the hands and wrists as well as mild sclerodactyly and difficulty swallowing solid foods. Laboratory studies reveal a positive serum antinuclear antibody assay at a dilution of 1:160. The most likely diagnosis of this woman's disorder is

(A) dermatomyositis

(B) mixed connective-tissue disease

(C) overlap syndrome

(D) systemic lupus erythematosus

(E) systemic sclerosis

108. A 26-year-old woman has painful mouth ulcers. Six weeks ago, she was started on propylthiouracil for hyperthyroidism. She is afebrile, and physical examination is unremarkable except for several small oral aphthous ulcers. White blood cell count is 200/mm^3 (15 percent neutrophils, 80 percent lymphocytes, 5 percent monocytes); hemoglobin concentration, hematocrit, and platelet count are normal. The woman's physician should stop the propylthiouracil and

(A) schedule a follow-up outpatient appointment

(B) arrange for HLA typing of her siblings in preparation for bone marrow transplantation

(C) prescribe oral prednisone, 1 mg/kg

(D) hospitalize her for broad-spectrum antibiotic therapy

(E) hospitalize her for white blood cell transfusion

109. Concerning a patient with adenocarcinoma of the pancreas, which of the following statements is true?

(A) It occurs most frequently in the body of the gland

(B) It carries a 22 percent 5-year survival rate

(C) It is nonresectable if it presents as painless jaundice

(D) It is associated with diabetes mellitus

(E) Tumors in the tail of the gland tend to be resectable

110. Pregnant women who have diabetes mellitus are affected more often than nondiabetic women by which of the following conditions?

(A) Hydramnios

(B) Infection

(C) Postpartum hemorrhage after vaginal delivery

(D) Preeclampsia and eclampsia

(E) All of the above

111. A 45-year-old woman with long-standing rheumatoid arthritis is diagnosed as having "anemia of chronic disease." The predominant mechanism causing this type of anemia in persons with chronic inflammatory disorders is

(A) defective porphyrin synthesis

(B) impaired incorporation of iron into porphyrin

(C) intravascular hemolysis

(D) depressed erythroid maturation due to decreased erythropoietin production

(E) impaired transfer of reticuloendothelial storage iron to marrow erythroid precursors

112. A 16-year-old boy presented with deep vein thrombophlebitis and pulmonary embolism. There is no familial history of thromboembolic disease. The platelet count on admission was 325,000/mm^3; prothrombin time, 13.1 s (control 11.4 s); partial thromboplastin time, 55.0 s (control 27.9 s); and thrombin time, 14.5 s (control 15 s). The most likely reason for the thrombotic diathesis in this patient is the presence of

(A) congenital antithrombin III deficiency
(B) dysfibrinogenemia
(C) factor XI deficiency
(D) lupus anticoagulant
(E) protein C deficiency

---

113. Which of the following groups would be most likely to develop acute leukemia?

(A) Persons who have Wiskott-Aldrich syndrome
(B) Persons who have hereditary sideroblastic anemia
(C) Persons who have paroxysmal nocturnal hemoglobinuria
(D) Persons who have Hodgkin's disease and are treated with radiation therapy
(E) Persons receiving immunosuppressive therapy following renal transplantation

114. Which of the following studies would be most useful to confirm the diagnosis in a patient with a skin lesion suggestive of Lyme disease?

(A) Skin biopsy
(B) Giemsa or Wright stain of a blood smear
(C) Culture of skin or blood in Kelly's modified medium
(D) Acute and convalescent serologic studies after several weeks of symptoms
(E) Examination of cerebrospinal fluid

115. A 50-year-old woman presents with fever, abdominal cramps, and watery diarrhea 1 week after finishing an oral course of ampicillin for cystitis. The best way to document pseudomembranous colitis caused by *Clostridium difficile* is

(A) stool culture
(B) a rise in serologic titers to *C. difficile*
(C) the presence of characteristic pseudomembranes on endoscopy
(D) cytopathic effect of stool filtrate on tissue culture monolayers
(E) Gram stain of the stool showing sheets of neutrophils and gram-positive rods

116. Which of the following statements is true regarding villous adenomas?

(A) These tumors are usually small (less than 3 cm) when initially diagnosed
(B) The malignant potential is lower than with tubular adenomas
(C) They are more frequently encountered in the proximal colon than in the rectosigmoid colon
(D) They are the hereditary polyps seen in familial colonic polyposis
(E) They are often sessrle and may not be amenable to colonoscopic removal

DIRECTIONS (Questions 117-120): Each question below contains five suggested responses. Select the **EXACT** number of responses indicated by each question.

117. Select the characteristics associated with Lambert-Eaton syndrome.
(SELECT 3 CHARACTERISTICS)

(A) Autonomic changes such as impotence or dry mouth

(B) Hyperreflexia

(C) Impaired acetylcholine release

(D) Predisposes to underlying malignancy

(E) Proximal muscle weakness

118. Despite optimal anti-ulcer therapy, a 32-year-old male has persistent peptic ulceration. You suspect that he may have Zollinger-Ellison syndrome. Which of the following statements are true regarding the Zollinger-Ellison syndrome?
(SELECT 2 STATEMENTS)

(A) The pancreatic islet cell tumor associated with this condition is the gastrinoma

(B) Gastrinomas are usually solitary and seldom malignant

(C) Optimal treatment is now thought to be complete gastrectomy and vagotomy

(D) When associated with parathyroid and pituitary tumors, multiple endocrine neoplasia I (MEN I) should be suspected

(E) Most frequently, these patients will have multiple post-bulbar duodenal ulcerations

Questions 119-120: A 53-year-old white female presents to your office with the referral diagnosis of myasthenia gravis. You suspect she has a dystrophic muscular disorder.

119. Which of the following is the most likely diagnosis in this patient?
(SELECT 1 CHOICE)

(A) Duchenne's dystrophy

(B) Facioscapulohumeral dystrophy

(C) Limb-girdle dystrophy

(D) Myotonic dystrophy

(E) Oculopharyngeal dystrophy

120. Which of the following support your diagnosis?
(SELECT 3 SIGNS OR SYMPTOMS)

(A) Aspiration pneumonia

(B) Foot-drop

(C) Neck muscle weakness

(D) Progressive external ophthalmoplegia

(E) Siblings unaffected by this disease

DIRECTIONS (Questions 121-137): Each **NEGATIVELY** phrased question below contains four or five suggested responses. Select the **one best** response to each question.

121. Legionnaire's disease is characterized by all of the following statements EXCEPT

(A) The disease is not spread from person to person

(B) Diarrhea, nausea, and vomiting often are prominent early symptoms

(C) Chest x-ray usually shows few abnormalities, while chest examination usually is markedly abnormal

(D) Fever is usually prolonged

(E) Therapy with erythromycin is recommended

122. A 58-year-old schoolteacher is hospitalized after 10 days of a respiratory illness. For 2 days he has had a dramatically worsening cough and shortness of breath. He also has had severe malaise, myalgias, arthralgias, rhinorrhea, and pharyngitis and has lost 2.7 kg (6 lb). No sputum or respiratory secretions can be collected. Chest x-ray shows a diffuse bronchopneumonia. All the following antibiotics would be acceptable for the initial treatment of this man's illness EXCEPT

(A) cephalothin

(B) clindamycin

(C) nafcillin

(D) penicillin G

(E) vancomycin

123. Acyclovir is indicated for treatment of all of the following EXCEPT

(A) chronic suppression of frequently recurring genital herpes

(B) herpes encephalitis

(C) herpes zoster in elderly patients to prevent dissemination and postherpetic neuralgia

(D) mucocutaneous herpes infection in immunocompromised patients

(E) prophylactically to prevent herpes infection during periods of immunosuppression

124. While treating a 67-year-old cardiac patient, it is necessary to lower his plasma potassium level. Which of the following agents would be LEAST effective in lowering his potassium level?

(A) Calcium gluconate

(B) Glucose and insulin

(C) Sodium bicarbonate

(D) Sodium polystyrene sulfonate (Kayexalate)

125. A 26-year-old man has substernal pleuritic chest pain that improves markedly when he sits upright. An EKG shows diffuse ST-segment elevation. Which of the following EKG changes LEAST supports a diagnosis of acute pericarditis?

(A) Frequent atrial premature beats

(B) PR-segment depression

(C) Diffuse T-wave inversion with ST-segment elevation

(D) Twice-normal serum creatine phosphokinase concentration

(E) No rub

126. All of the following statements concerning a hysterosalpingogram test for fallopian-tube patency are true EXCEPT

(A) the contrast medium used should be either oil- or water-soluble

(B) salpingitis isthmica nodosa may be diagnosed with this procedure

(C) uterine cavity abnormalities (i.e., polyps, adhesions) may be diagnosed with this procedure

(D) less than 3 mL of contrast medium should be used to avoid spill from the tubes into the peritoneal cavity

(E) the test has been shown to have a therapeutic effect in some cases of infertility

127. Which of the following tests is NOT helpful in the diagnosis of an ectopic pregnancy?

(A) Abdominal flat plate

(B) Culdocentesis

(C) Pelvic examination

(D) Pregnancy test

(E) Ultrasound

128. Elements that a plaintiff must prove in a malpractice action in establishing the standard of care include all of the following EXCEPT

(A) the defendant owed a duty to the patient

(B) the defendant breached a duty to the patient

(C) the breach caused damage to the plaintiff

(D) the duty is to give the best care possible in the given field

129. Asherman syndrome is associated with infertility. All of the following are true EXCEPT

(A) symptoms include amenorrhea or hypomenorrhea

(B) patients are usually anovulatory

(C) diagnosis can be made by hysterosalpingogram

(D) treatment consists of lysis of adhesions

(E) prophylactic antibiotics are a wise precaution for the surgical treatment of Asherman syndrome

130. Which of the following vaccines is NOT recommended for use in immunocompromised adults?

(A) Bacille Calmette-Guerin (BCG) vaccine (against tuberculosis)

(B) Inactivated influenza vaccine for current year

(C) 23-Valent pneumococcal vaccine

(D) Quadrivalent meningococcal vaccine

(E) Inactivated polio vaccine

131. The intramuscular administration of RH_0 immunoglobulin is recommended in all of the following situations EXCEPT

(A) all Rh-negative, nonsensitized women at 28 to 32 weeks of gestation

(B) all Rh-negative, nonsensitized women within 72 h of the birth of an Rh-positive infant

(C) after an episode of uterine bleeding in an Rh-negative, nonsensitized woman

(D) after amniocentesis in an Rh-negative, sensitized woman

132. Which of the following statements regarding percutaneous transluminal coronary angioplasty (PTCA) is NOT correct?

(A) Restenosis resulting after successful dilation develops in approximately 20 percent of patients within 6 months

(B) Stenoses within saphenous vein bypass grafts can be dilated using this technique

(C) A recent complete occlusion of a coronary artery can be successfully dilated using this technique

(D) A 65 percent stenosis of the left main coronary artery is a contraindication to this procedure

(E) If restenosis develops several weeks after a successful dilation, repeated PTCA is unlikely to be successful

133. Which of the following physical findings is NOT seen in osteoarthritis?

(A) Bony crepitus on joint movement

(B) Bouchard's nodes

(C) Boutonnière deformity

(D) Heberden's nodes

(E) Positive "shrug" sign

134. Which of the following conditions is NOT usually associated with a megaloblastic anemia?

(A) Alcoholism

(B) Non-tropical sprue

(C) Pregnancy

(D) Total gastrectomy

(E) Zollinger-Ellison syndrome

135. Which of the following factors is NOT thought to contribute to the pathogenicity of staphylococci?

(A) Catalase production

(B) Coagulase production

(C) Enterotoxin production

(D) Exotoxin production

(E) Penicillinase production

136. The association of low maternal serum alpha-fetoprotein values and increased risk of chromosomal abnormalities, most notably Down syndrome, has been known for a number of years. Which of the following factors does NOT affect the determination of the multiple of the median for maternal serum alpha-fetoprotein values?

(A) Gestational age

(B) Maternal age

(C) Maternal weight

(D) Multiple gestations

(E) Race

137. A 33-year-old woman presents with pain in her right wrist. The pain first appeared when she was pregnant with her third child and has recurred more or less monthly for the last six months since she delivered. A neurologist has diagnosed carpal tunnel syndrome. Which of the following statements regarding the carpal tunnel syndrome is NOT correct?

(A) It is often secondary to a wrist fracture

(B) It may be associated with pregnancy

(C) It may cause nocturnal dysesthesia

(D) It is often associated with vascular compromise

(E) It is often associated with the menstrual cycle

DIRECTIONS (Questions 138-200): Each set of matching questions in this section consists of a list of four to twenty-six lettered options followed by numbered questions. For each numbered question, select the appropriate lettered option(s). Each lettered option may be used **once, more than once, or not at all.** The question will state the **EXACT NUMBER** of options to select.

Questions 138-139: Match each of the numbered characteristics with the renal tumors listed below.

(A) Angiomyolipoma

(B) Lymphoma

(C) Oncocytoma

(D) Wilm's tumor

138. Favorable vs. unfavorable histology **(SELECT 1 TUMOR)**

139. Tuberous sclerosis **(SELECT 1 TUMOR)**

Questions 140-141: Match the numbered type of renal stone with the appropriate treatment.

(A) Allopurinol

(B) Antibiotics

(C) Fluids, alkalinization

(D) Thiazide diuretics

140. Struvite **(SELECT 1 TREATMENT)**

141. Uric acid **(SELECT 1 TREATMENT)**

Questions 142-143: Match the side effects below with the appropriate anesthetic.

(A) Enflurane

(B) Halothane

(C) Methoxyflurane

(D) Morphine

(E) Nitrous oxide (N_2O)

142. Decreased peripheral resistance **(SELECT 1 ANESTHETIC)**

143. Possible worsening of distention in bowel obstruction **(SELECT 1 ANESTHETIC)**

Questions 144-146: A teenager with new onset seizures is to begin anticonvulsant therapy. She has concerns about potential side effects. For each systemic side effect listed below, choose the anticonvulsant drug with which it is most likely to be associated.

(A) Carbamazepine

(B) Clonazepam

(C) Phenobarbital

(D) Phenytoin

(E) Valproic acid

144. Osteomalacia **(SELECT 1 DRUG)**

145. Lymphadenopathy **(SELECT 1 DRUG)**

146. Acute hepatic failure **(SELECT 1 DRUG)**

Questions 147-148: For each description below, select the type of fracture or dislocation with which is it most likely to be associated.

(A) Greenstick fracture

(B) Monteggia's deformity

(C) Navicular fracture

(D) Posterior shoulder dislocation

(E) Spiral fracture

147. Dislocation of the radial head and fracture of the proximal third of the ulna
(SELECT 1 CHOICE)

148. Tenderness in the anatomical snuffbox
(SELECT 1 CHOICE)

Questions 149-150: Match each of the numbered chemotherapeutic agents to its appropriate mechanism of action.

(A) Binds with DNA and causes untwisting of the double helix

(B) Blocks thymidylate synthetase

(C) Causes depurination and miscoding errors by its alkylating action

(D) Inhibits DNA synthesis and reacts with DNA to cause strand scission

(E) Produces metaphase arrest by direct binding to tubulin

149. Vinblastine
(SELECT 1 MECHANISM)

150. 5-Fluorouracil
(SELECT 1 MECHANISM)

Questions 151-153: For each of the disorders below, select the characteristic hemodynamic pattern.

(A) Dip-and-plateau pattern

(B) Equalization of diastolic pressures

(C) Slow *y* descent

(D) Tall *v* wave

(E) None of the above

151. Mitral stenosis
(SELECT 1 PATTERN)

152. Acute mitral regurgitation
(SELECT 1 PATTERN)

153. Acute septal rupture
(SELECT 1 PATTERN)

Questions 154-155: Match each numbered drug or characteristic with the appropriate form of esophagitis.

(A) *Candida*

(B) *Herpes simplex* virus

(C) Pill-induced

(D) Radiation

154. Cyclophosphamide
(SELECT 1 CHOICE)

155. Nodular filling defects
(SELECT 1 CHOICE)

Questions 156-157: Match the following pancreatic endocrine tumors with the clinical features below.

(A) Beta cell tumor

(B) Cholera-like symptoms

(C) Delta cell tumor

(D) Hyperglycemia

(E) Wheezing

156. Glucagonoma **(SELECT 1 FEATURE)**

157. VIPoma **(SELECT 1 FEATURE)**

Questions 158-159: Match each defect in host immunity with the type of infection most commonly associated with it.

(A) Cytomegalovirus

(B) Gram-negative bacteremia

(C) Recurrent *Neisseria gonorrhoeae* infections

(D) Recurrent staphylococcal skin abscesses

(E) *Streptococcus pneumoniae* bacteremia

158. Abnormal T-cell suppressor/helper ratio in patients with the acquired immunodeficiency syndrome (AIDS) **(SELECT 1 TYPE)**

159. Chédiak-Higashi syndrome **(SELECT 1 TYPE)**

Questions 160-161: For each of the numbered patients below, select the ultrasonic finding of most concern.

(A) Fetal ascites

(B) Malposition of the placenta

(C) Short femur length

(D) Spinal defects

(E) Twins

160. A patient is Rh-sensitized and has had a previous stillbirth **(SELECT 1 FINDING)**

161. A patient is referred for an ultrasound because of two elevated serum alpha-fetoprotein levels **(SELECT 1 FINDING)**

Questions 162-163: For each syndrome below, select the associated cardiovascular abnormality.

(A) Coarctation of the aorta

(B) Cor pulmonale

(C) Endocardial cushion defect

(D) Mitral regurgitation

(E) Pulmonic stenosis

162. Congenital rubella **(SELECT 1 ABNORMALITY)**

163. Cystic fibrosis **(SELECT 1 ABNORMALITY)**

Questions 164-165: Match the following numbered red blood cell morphologies with the associated disorder.

(A) Auto-immune hemolytic anemia

(B) Prosthetic heart valve

(C) Severe liver disease

(D) Thalassemia

164. Spherocytes **(SELECT 1 DISORDER)**

165. Target cells **(SELECT 1 DISORDER)**

Questions 166-167: Match each of the numbered malignancies with the appropriate cells or cellular characteristics.

(A) Cytoplasmic extensions

(B) Langerhans' cells

(C) Osteoclast activating factor

(D) Reed-Sternberg cells

166. Hodgkin's disease **(SELECT 1 CHOICE)**

167. Histiocytosis **(SELECT 1 CHOICE)**

Questions 168-169: Match each of the numbered causes of right heart failure below with the most characteristic set of hemodynamic measurements.

	Right atrial pressure, mmHg	Pulmonary arterial pressure, mmHg	Pulmonary capillary wedge pressure, mmHg
(A)	16	75/30	11
(B)	16	35/17	16
(C)	16	100/30	28
(D)	16	45/22	20
(E)	16	22/12	10
Normal values	0-5	12-28/3-13	3-11

168. Mitral stenosis **(SELECT 1 SET OF MEASUREMENTS)**

169. Constrictive pericarditis **(SELECT 1 SET OF MEASUREMENTS)**

Questions 170-171: There are several mechanisms that affect blood clotting. Match the following tests with the coagulation mechanism they most specifically evaluate.

(A) Extrinsic pathway

(B) Fibrinogen function

(C) Intrinsic pathway

(D) Platelet function

(E) None of the above

170. Partial thromboplastin time **(SELECT 1 MECHANISM)**

171. Prothrombin time **(SELECT 1 MECHANISM)**

Questions 172-173: Match the following numbered hereditary syndromes with the associated tumors.

(A) Glioblastoma

(B) Leukemia

(C) Renal cell carcinoma

(D) Rhabdomyoma

172. Tuberous sclerosis
(SELECT 1 TUMOR)

173. von Hippel-Lindau
(SELECT 1 TUMOR)

Questions 174-176: For each description below, select the type of bone lesion with which it is most likely to be associated.

(A) Aneurysmal bone cyst

(B) Osteochondroma

(C) Osteoid osteoma

(D) Osteosarcoma

(E) Unicameral bone cyst

174. Arises from the cartilaginous elements of developing bone; frequently asymptomatic
(SELECT 1 LESION)

175. X-ray may show a round or oval defect in the bone without adjacent reactive bone formation; the most common presenting symptom is pathologic fracture
(SELECT 1 LESION)

176. Proliferation of vascular tissue in bone destroys the overlying bone cortex
(SELECT 1 LESION)

Questions 177-178: Match each numbered description with the correct type of abortion.

(A) Complete abortion

(B) Incomplete abortion

(C) Inevitable abortion

(D) Missed abortion

(E) Threatened abortion

177. Uterine bleeding at 7 weeks' gestation without any cervical dilation
(SELECT 1 CHOICE)

178. Expulsion of all fetal and placental tissue from the uterine cavity at 10 weeks' gestation **(SELECT 1 CHOICE)**

Questions 179-180: For each of the numbered syndromes or diseases below, choose the virus responsible when the fetus is exposed in utero.

(A) Cytomegalovirus

(B) Hepatitis B

(C) Rubella

(D) Rubeola

(E) Varicella zoster

179. Cicatricial skin lesions, limb hypoplasia, rudimentary digits **(SELECT 1 VIRUS)**

180. Microcephaly, intracerebral calcifications, hepatosplenomegaly **(SELECT 1 VIRUS)**

Questions 181-182: Match the following numbered polyposis syndromes to their corresponding feature.

(A) Adenoma

(B) Brain tumors

(C) Hamartoma

(D) Osteomas

181. Peutz-Jeghers **(SELECT 1 FEATURE)**

182. Turcot's **(SELECT 1 FEATURE)**

Questions 183-184: Match the descriptions below with the appropriate infectious agent or condition.

(A) Atrophic (senile) vaginitis

(B) *Candida albicans*

(C) *Gardnerella vaginalis* (formerly *Haemophilus vaginalis*)

(D) *Neisseria gonorrhoeae*

(E) *Trichomonas vaginalis*

183. Typically produces a grossly recognizable vaginal mucosa with punctate hemorrhage ("strawberry spots") **(SELECT 1 CHOICE)**

184. Treatment with an estrogen cream may be effective **(SELECT 1 CHOICE)**

Questions 185-186: Match the gastrointestinal content at each site with its appropriate ionic composition (meq/L).

	Na^+	K^+	Cl^-	HCO_3^-
(A)	140	5	104	30
(B)	140	5	75	115
(C)	60	10	130	0
(D)	10	26	10	30
(E)	60	30	40	50

185. Small bowel **(SELECT 1 IONIC COMPOSITION)**

186. Colon **(SELECT 1 IONIC COMPOSITION)**

Questions 187-188: Match the numbered hepatobiliary abnormality with the most appropriate nuclear medicine study listed below.

(A) Iminoacetic acid cholecystectomy

(B) Labeled red blood cells (RBCs)

(C) Sulfur colloid

(D) Xenon

187. Fatty liver **(SELECT 1 STUDY)**

188. Focal nodular hyperplasia (FNH) **(SELECT 1 STUDY)**

Questions 189-190: Match each of the following complications to the disease with which it is most commonly associated.

(A) AIDS

(B) Histiocytosis X

(C) Hodgkin disease

(D) Mucocutaneous lymph node syndrome

(E) Varicella infection

189. Coronary artery aneurysm **(SELECT 1 DISEASE)**

190. Lymphocytic interstitial pneumonitis **(SELECT 1 DISEASE)**

Questions 191-192: For each radiologic or angiographic sign or characteristic, select the cardiovascular anomaly with which it is most closely associated.

(A) Egg on its side or egg on a string

(B) Figure eight or snowman

(C) Goetz sign

(D) Gooseneck deformity

(E) Waterfall pulmonary hilum

191. Single ventricle with transposition of the great vessels **(SELECT 1 ANOMALY)**

192. Supracardiac total anomalous pulmonary venous return **(SELECT 1 ANOMALY)**

Questions 193-195: Match the numbered chemotherapeutic agents with their most common side effects.

(A) Cardiac toxicity

(B) Hemorrhagic cystitis

(C) Necrotizing enterocolitis

(D) Ocular degeneration

(E) Pancreatic failure

(F) Peripheral neuropathy

(G) Pulmonary fibrosis

(H) Renal failure

(I) Tympanic membrane fibrosis

193. Bleomycin **(SELECT 1 SIDE EFFECT)**

194. Doxorubicin **(SELECT 1 SIDE EFFECT)**

195. Vincristine **(SELECT 1 SIDE EFFECT)**

Questions 196-198: Match each numbered type of azotemia with the following conditions or drugs associated with it.

(A) Crush injury

(B) Cirrhosis

(C) Cyclooxygenase inhibitors

(D) Gentamycin

(E) Methicillin

(F) Myeloma

(G) Retroperitoneal fibrosis

(H) Severe burns

(I) Straddle injury

196. Prerenal
(SELECT 1 CONDITION OR DRUG)

197. Renal
(SELECT 4 CONDITIONS OR DRUGS)

198. Postrenal
(SELECT 2 CONDITIONS OR DRUGS)

Questions 199-200: Match the numbered diseases with the following lettered features.

(A) Benign pneumoperitoneum

(B) Biliary tract disease

(C) Continuous involvement of the colon

(D) Fistula

(E) Granulomas

(F) Increased incidence in Jews

(G) Prophylactic colectomy

(H) Rectal disease

(I) Transmural inflammation

199. Ulcerative colitis
(SELECT 5 FEATURES)

200. Crohn's disease
(SELECT 6 FEATURES)

STOP. You have completed this section of the PreTest Examination. Go back over your answers and be sure your answer sheet is carefully marked. Do not apply any remaining time from this section to the second section of this PreTest.

Book B

Time: Three hours and thirty minutes

Number of items: 200

Book B

DIRECTIONS (Questions 201-321): Each question below contains four or five suggested responses. Select the **one best** response to each question.

201. A 22-year-old patient with cystic fibrosis presents to the emergency room with new onset hemoptysis. Which of the following statements is true?

(A) Small volume hemoptysis is rarely seen in these patients

(B) Large volume hemoptysis is likely due to bronchial artery bleeding

(C) Single-drug antibiotic therapy is preferred to a multi-drug regimen to decrease the development of drug-resistant microbes

(D) It is likely that the patient had meconium ileus as a neonate

(E) The development of digital clubbing is uncommon with late stage cystic fibrosis for unknown reasons

202. Which of the following statements concerning intussusception in infants is correct?

(A) Recurrence rates following treatment are greater than 20 percent

(B) It is frequently preceded by a gastrointestinal viral illness

(C) A 1- to 2-week period of parenteral alimentation should precede surgical reduction when surgery is required

(D) Pneumatic reduction without surgery is not appropriate in this case

(E) Colocolic intussusceptions are the most common

Questions 203-204: A patient recently underwent surgery for carcinoma of the hepatic flexure and required prolonged nasogastric intubation. The following laboratory values were obtained:

Arterial blood gases:
pH 7.56; P_{O_2} 85 torr; P_{CO_2} 50 torr

Serum electrolytes (meq/L):
Na^+ 132; K^+ 3.1; Cl^- 80; HCO_3^- 42

Urine electrolytes (meq/L):
Na^+ 2; K^- 5; Cl^- 6

203. Based on these laboratory values, the best descriptive diagnosis is

(A) combined metabolic alkalosis

(B) metabolic alkalosis with respiratory compensation

(C) mixed respiratory acidosis with metabolic compensation

(D) "paradoxical" metabolic respiratory alkalosis

(E) pure metabolic alkalosis

204. The most appropriate therapy for this patient is

(A) administration of acetazolamide to promote renal excretion of bicarbonate

(B) clamping the nasogastric tube to prevent further acid losses

(C) infusion of 0.9 percent NaCl with supplemental KCl

(D) infusion of isotonic (0.15 *N*) HCl via a central venous catheter

(E) intubation and controlled hypoventilation on a volume-cycled ventilator to further increase the P_{CO_2}

205. The most common abnormality of the adrenogenital syndrome is

(A) 11-hydroxylase deficiency

(B) 17-hydroxylase deficiency

(C) 21-hydroxylase excess

(D) 21-hydroxylase deficiency

(E) 3-beta-ol-dehydrogenase deficiency

206. Four days after a cadaveric renal allograft, a 26-year-old female with diabetic nephropathy has a serum creatinine concentration of 160 μmol/L (1.8 mg/dL). She is being treated with cyclosporine and prednisone. Urine output decreases and serum creatinine increases. Blood pressure and temperature are unremarkable. The best initial step in management would be to

(A) administer an intravenous bolus of furosemide

(B) administer pulsed steroid therapy

(C) decrease the dose of cyclosporine

(D) obtain a biopsy of the renal allograft

(E) obtain ultrasonography of the renal allograft

207. Which of the following statements is true regarding bladder cancer?

(A) Histologically, squamous cell carcinoma is far more common than transitional cell carcinoma

(B) Ureteral obstruction is common

(C) Squamous cell carcinoma is more common in Egypt than in North America

(D) Pelvic pain is the most common presenting symptom

208. The chest radiograph shown is that of a 65-year-old man with slowly progressive shortness of breath.

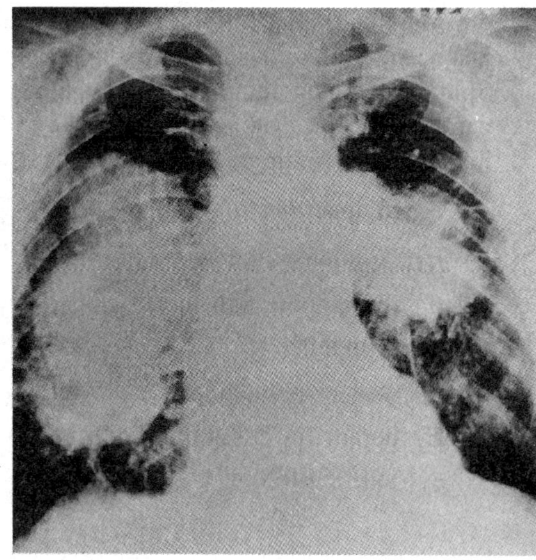

Which of the following is the most likely diagnosis?

(A) Sarcoidosis

(B) Bilateral bronchogenic carcinoma

(C) Echinococcal disease

(D) Wegener granulomatosis

(E) Progressive massive fibrosis

209. A woman who has rheumatoid arthritis suddenly develops pain and swelling in the right calf. The most likely diagnosis is

(A) Achilles tendonitis

(B) deep thrombophlebitis

(C) pes anserinus bursitis

(D) ruptured plantaris tendon

(E) ruptured popliteal cyst

210. During a routine physical examination of a 59-year-old man with long-standing rheumatoid arthritis, a 2.5-cm pulmonary nodule and ipsilateral hilar lymphadenopathy are observed on routine chest x-ray. The patient has been a smoker since he was in his teens. Sputum cytology demonstrates squamous carcinoma cells. The most appropriate management would be

(A) an upper gastrointestinal series

(B) exploratory thoracotomy

(C) observation with chest x-rays every 4 months

(D) scalene node biopsy

(E) therapy for 2 months with oral corticosteroids

211. A 68-year-old, previously healthy woman develops a lilac-colored rash in a butterfly distribution about the eyes, on the bridge of the nose, and on the cheeks. She has a similar rash on her knuckles. She has had an associated muscle weakness manifested by difficulty arising from a chair or climbing stairs. She takes no medicines. Other than the rash and proximal muscle weakness, the woman's examination is unremarkable. The most appropriate subsequent procedure would be

(A) barium enema, upper-GI series, intravenous pyelography, mammography, and chest x-ray

(B) biopsy of an affected muscle

(C) electromyography (EMG)

(D) glucocorticoid treatment

(E) hemogram, serum chemistries, Pap smear, urinalysis, mammography, and chest x-ray

212. Over the course of the last year, a 55-year-old man has experienced vague postprandial epigastric fullness. He initially treated himself with antacids without success. For the last several months, he has been anorectic and has lost 4.5 kg (10 lb). Physical examination is unrevealing except for faintly guaiac-positive stool. Hematocrit is 26 percent. A representative x-ray from his upper gastrointestinal series is reproduced below.

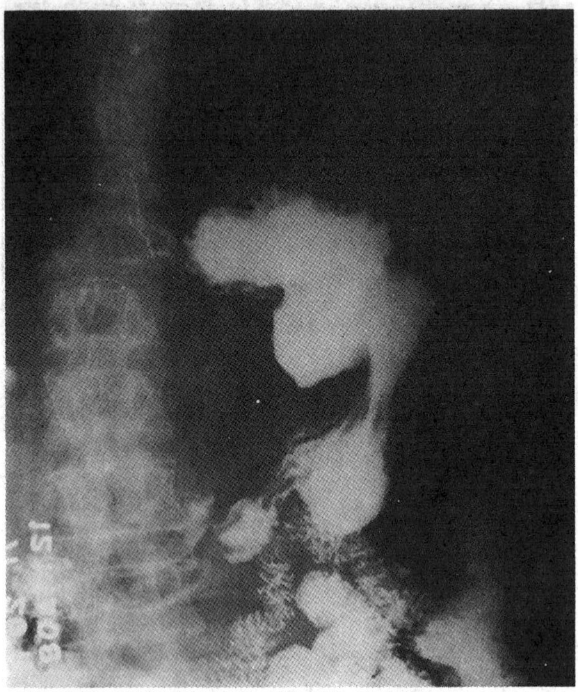

The man's physician should now

(A) perform a double-contrast upper gastrointestinal series

(B) perform gastroscopy

(C) prescribe cimetidine

(D) prescribe metoclopramide

(E) recommend total gastrectomy

213. A 42-year-old woman is concerned that she may be having "hot flashes." Her menses are less frequent and the amount of menstrual flow is unpredictable. The most accurate indicator of primary ovarian failure in this case would be a serum level of

(A) estrone < 20 pg/mL

(B) prolactin > 10 ng/mL

(C) androstenedione > 600 pg/mL

(D) luteinizing hormones > 30 mIU/mL

(E) follicle-stimulating hormones > 40 mIU/mL

214. You have been caring for a 67-year-old patient with squamous cell carcinoma of the lung. Upon examination, you note muscle wasting. Underlying causes may be due to which of the following?

(A) Cachexia

(B) Paraneoplastic neuropathy

(C) Polymyositis

(D) Type II fiber atrophy

(E) All of the above

215. Which of the following cells produce follicle-stimulating hormone?

(A) Acidophilic cells of the adenohypophysis

(B) Basophilic cells of the adenohypophysis

(C) Chromophobe cells of the adenohypophysis

(D) Theca interna cells

(E) None of the above

216. What is the most common malignant tumor of the liver?

(A) Angiosarcoma

(B) Cavernous hemangioma

(C) Hamartoma

(D) Hepatocellular carcinoma

(E) Metastatic neoplasms

Questions 217-218: Following an automobile accident, a 4-year-old boy is brought to the emergency room. Upon examination, he is found to have fractures of the 10th and 11th ribs on the left side and a falling hematocrit.

217. Which organ is most likely to have been injured following the blunt trauma to this patient's abdomen and may be causing the internal bleeding?

(A) Intestine

(B) Kidney

(C) Liver

(D) Pancreas

(E) Spleen

218. Because of evidence of continuing bleeding, the patient is taken to the operating room where abdominal exploration discloses a laceration of the lower pole of the spleen. The surgeon should

(A) ligate the splenic artery but **leave the** spleen in place

(B) perform splenectomy

(C) perform a partial splenectomy

(D) perform a splenorrhaphy (repair of the laceration)

(E) cauterize the spleen and place a drain in the area

219. A 27-year-old man seeks advice because he has noticed fasciculations in his calf muscles. He has no other complaints. Examination shows that muscle bulk and strength, tendon and plantar reflexes, and sensory function are all normal. He should undergo

(A) electromyography

(B) muscle biopsy

(C) myelography

(D) sural nerve biopsy

(E) none of the above

220. At laparotomy, an irregular uterus with wormlike extension in the veins is seen. This finding, together with red staining cells found within vessels of the myometrium, is consistent with

(A) adenomyosis

(B) endometriosis

(C) intravenous leiomyomatosis

(D) endolymphatic stromal myosis

(E) uterine sarcoma

221. A 53-year-old hypertensive man develops right hemiparesis. He has no sensory changes, papilledema, or aphasia. A CT scan performed several days after gathering this information would most likely reveal

(A) atrophy

(B) large infarction in the left cerebral cortex

(C) left cerebral cortical hemorrhage

(D) right internal capsule hemorrhage

(E) small infarction in the left internal capsule

222. The weakness associated with myasthenia gravis is due to which of the following disorders in the neuromuscular junction?

(A) Damage of postsynaptic membranes by T lymphocytes

(B) Degradation and blockage of postsynaptic receptors

(C) Presence of antibodies against presynaptic membranes

(D) Presynaptic block in release of acetylcholine

(E) Reduced acetylcholine in presynaptic vesicles

223. The most common etiologic process in the development of pyogenic liver abscess is

(A) appendicitis

(B) cholangitis

(C) diverticulitis

(D) generalized sepsis

(E) hepatic trauma

224. A 60-year-old, mildly obese woman complains of a very bothersome burning pain on the anterolateral aspect of her right thigh from the groin almost as far distally as the knee. Examination shows reduction of sensation to touch and pinprick in the affected area. There is no loss of muscle strength and reflexes are normal. The most likely diagnosis is

(A) compression of the lateral femoral cutaneous nerve

(B) disruption of the lumbosacral plexus

(C) femoral hernia

(D) nutritional neuropathy

(E) ruptured intervertebral disk

Questions 225-226: Following a viral illness, a 27-year-old male presents to the emergency room with increasing weakness and fatigue. He is areflexic but has preserved sensory function. The working diagnosis is Guillain-Barré syndrome.

225. Which of the following pathologic findings supports this diagnosis?

(A) Destruction of axons

(B) Inflammation of sensory ganglia

(C) Loss of anterior horn cells

(D) Segmental demyelination

(E) Wallerian degeneration

226. Which statement is true regarding Guillain-Barré syndrome?

(A) Complete recovery is likely

(B) Plasmaphoresis should be instituted routinely

(C) Corticosteroids are effective in reducing the need for ventilatory support

(D) There are marked variations in the incidence of Guillain-Barré syndrome worldwide

(E) Herpes infections account for only a small proportion of those cases thought to be associated with viruses

227. Which of the following findings is most commonly associated with idiopathic retroperitoneal fibrosis?

(A) Calf claudication

(B) Intestinal obstruction

(C) Jaundice

(D) Leg edema

(E) Ureteral obstruction

228. A 35-year-old woman, who has signs and symptoms of mitral stenosis, is found to have a 3-cm tumor in the left atrium. This mass is most likely to be a

(A) hemangioma

(B) malignant lymphoma

(C) metastatic carcinoma

(D) myxoma

(E) rhabdomyoma

Questions 229-230: You have been caring for a 58-year-old man for the past 10 years. He was formerly an active alcoholic but has been sober for 8 years. He now has progressive dysarthria, tongue dystonia, shuffling gait, and fast tremor that worsens as his hand moves toward a target.

229. The disease process causing these symptoms most likely is

(A) acquired hepatocerebral degeneration

(B) Marchiafava-Bignami disease

(C) paracarcinomatous syndrome

(D) Wernicke's disease

(E) Wilson's disease

230. The single most appropriate imaging study in this patient is which of the following?

(A) Contrast-enhanced cranial CT

(B) Skull series with special views of the mastoid air cells

(C) Magnetic resonance imaging (MRI) with magnetic resonance angiography

(D) Transfemoral cerebral angiography

(E) ^{99m}Tc-glucoheptonate brain scan with SPECT imaging

231. A 19-year-old college student presents to the college health service with a four-day history of back pain in the midlumbar area, difficulty in starting urination, and paresthesias in the feet. She is febrile, physical exam with straight leg raising produces pain, slight hip weakness is present, and Babinski signs are absent. The physician should

(A) arrange for emergency MRI of the spine

(B) obtain blood cultures and start antibiotic therapy

(C) obtain spine films and a bone scan

(D) obtain urinalysis and abdominal plain films

(E) perform a lumbar puncture

232. For the last 5 weeks, a 35-year-old woman has had episodes of intense vertigo lasting several hours. Each episode is associated with tinnitus and a sense of fullness in her right ear; during the attacks, she prefers to lie on her left side. Examination during an attack shows that she has fine rotatory nystagmus, which is maximal on gaze to the left. There are no ocular palsies, cranial-nerve signs, or long-tract signs. An audiogram shows a high-tone hearing loss in the right ear, with recruitment but no tone decay. The most likely diagnosis in the case described is

(A) acoustic neurinoma

(B) labyrinthitis

(C) Ménière's disease

(D) multiple sclerosis

(E) vertebral-basilar insufficiency

233. A 75-year-old woman has daily episodes of light-headedness. A rhythm strip obtained in the emergency room shows sinus bradycardia at 51 beats per minute and 2.8-second sinus pause that produces no symptoms. The next step in this woman's management should be

(A) implantation of a permanent demand ventricular pacemaker

(B) trial of a temporary transvenous pacemaker

(C) institution of sublingual isoproterenol therapy

(D) continuous 24-hour Holter monitoring

(E) exercise tolerance testing

234. A 60-year-old man is admitted to a hospital because of respiratory failure and tachycardia. His rectal temperature is 38.3°C (101°F), respiratory rate 32 breaths per minute, and blood pressure 100/60 mmHg. His admission electrocardiogram is shown below.

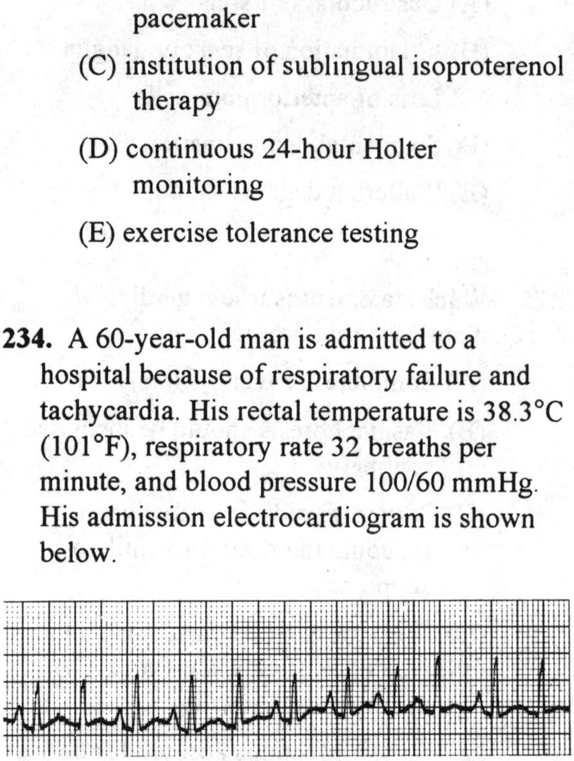

Which of the following measures would constitute the most appropriate management for this man?

(A) Electrical cardioversion after the blood pressure is raised

(B) Supplemental oxygenation or mechanical ventilation

(C) Administration of digitalis

(D) Administration of quinidine

(E) Administration of verapamil

235. You are called in to evaluate the heart of a 19-year-old primigravida at term. Which of the following auscultatory findings are considered normal changes for this pregnant patient?

(A) S_3

(B) Split S_2

(C) 2/6 systolic ejection murmur

(D) Soft diastolic murmur

(E) All of the above

236. A 67-year-old male presents with an insidious history of impotence and urinary incontinence. Physical findings include a tremor at rest, bradykinesia, rigidity, severe orthostatic hypotension, and anhidrosis. The most likely diagnosis is

(A) an autonomic form of the Landry-Guillain-Barré syndrome

(B) guanethidine intoxication

(C) micturition syncope

(D) Parkinson's disease

(E) the Shy-Drager syndrome

237. A 58-year-old male with long-standing essential hypertension presents with sudden onset of hemiplegia, slurred speech, and deviation of the eyes away from the side affected with hemiplegia. A hypertensive hemorrhage is suspected. The most common site for hypertensive brain hemorrhage is the

(A) central white matter

(B) cerebellar hemispheres

(C) pons

(D) putamen

(E) thalamus

Questions 238-239: A 27-year-old bisexual male is found to have mildly hyperdense solid tumors in the periventricular regions on cranial CT scanning.

238. The most likely diagnosis is

(A) B-cell lymphoma

(B) ependymoma

(C) glioblastoma

(D) medulloblastoma

(E) meningioma

239. Which of the following statements is true about this patient's tumor?

(A) It should respond well initially to chemotherapy and radiotherapy

(B) The overall prognosis is quite good with median survival approaching 10 years

(C) Surgical resection can be curative

(D) Spinal epidural lesions are seldom associated with this tumor

(E) This tumor is becoming increasingly uncommon

240. A 22-year-old woman, gravida 3, para 2 (one abortion), is brought to the hospital because she says she has been raped by a 35-year-old man whom she knows to have had a vasectomy two years ago. Both persons have an A-positive blood type. Which of the following would be most useful to her in the prosecution of this case?

(A) Accurate description of the introitus

(B) Examination of her pubic hair

(C) Smear for sperm from the cervix

(D) Specific typing of vaginal washings

(E) Vaginal washings for acid phosphatase

241. A 64-year-old man presents to the emergency room with large volume hematochezia. Which of the following disorders is the most likely source of massive bleeding from the lower gastrointestinal tract (distal to the ligament of Trietz)?

(A) Colonic carcinoma
(B) Diverticulitis
(C) Diverticulosis
(D) Meckel's diverticulum
(E) Ulcerative colitis

242. Hypertensive encephalopathy is characterized by which of the following?

(A) Disordered consciousness
(B) Papilledema
(C) Severe hypertension
(D) Seizures
(E) All of the above

243. A 61-year-old woman noticed severe sharp pain in her back after lifting a suitcase. A compression fracture of the T11 vertebral body is identified on x-ray examination. Routine laboratory evaluation discloses a serum calcium concentration of 2 mmol/L (8.0 mg/dL), a serum phosphorus concentration of 0.77 mmol/L (2.4 mg/dL), and increased serum alkaline phosphatase activity. The serum parathyroid hormone level was subsequently found to be elevated as well. The most likely diagnosis is

(A) ectopic parathyroid hormone secretion
(B) Paget's disease of bone
(C) postmenopausal osteoporosis
(D) primary hyperparathyroidism
(E) vitamin D deficiency

244. During a routine physical examination of a 7-year-old girl, you detect the beginning of pubertal changes. What is the most common cause of precocious puberty in girls?

(A) Albright syndrome
(B) Gonadal tumors
(C) Hypothyroidism
(D) No specific cause is identified; idiopathic
(E) Tumors of the central nervous system

245. A 12-year-old patient with absence seizures may manifest which of the following features?

(A) Present with an aura
(B) Have a characteristic electroencephalographic pattern
(C) Have many associated neurologic abnormalities
(D) Phenytoin is the drug of choice
(E) More than 90 percent of patients outgrow the condition

246. During a routine checkup, a 67-year-old man is found to have a level of serum alkaline phosphatase three times the upper limit of normal. Serum calcium and phosphorus concentrations and liver function test results are normal. He is asymptomatic. The most likely diagnosis is

(A) metastatic bone disease
(B) occult plasmacytoma
(C) osteomalacia
(D) Paget's disease of bone
(E) primary hyperparathyroidism

247. A 64-year-old man seeks medical attention because of an annoying cough. Physical examination is remarkable only for supraclavicular lymphadenopathy. Chest x-ray shows a parahilar mass and paratracheal lymph node enlargement. Serum and urine chemistries are as follows:

Sodium: 120 mmol/L
Potassium: 4 mmol/L
Bicarbonate: 23 mmol/L
Serum osmolality: 250 mosmol/kg H_2O
Urine osmolality: 600 mosmol/kg H_2O
Urine sodium: 80 mmol/L

The most likely pathophysiologic basis for this man's hyponatremia is

(A) production of a vasopressin-like molecule by tumor tissue

(B) production of authentic vasopressin by tumor tissue

(C) potentiation of vasopressin action on the renal tubule by a tumor product

(D) stimulation of neurohypophyseal vasopressin secretion by a tumor product

(E) central nervous system metastases resulting in loss of vasopressin regulation

248. A 55-year-old man presents to the emergency room with progressive dysphagia for the past year. He occasionally has regurgitated food particles eaten several days earlier. He notes that his breath has been foul-smelling. The most likely diagnosis is

(A) achalasia

(B) diabetic gastroparesis

(C) gastric outlet obstruction

(D) scleroderma

(E) Zenker's diverticulum

249. A 35-year-old female presents with renal calculi. You suspect she has primary hyperparathyroidism based on biochemical testing. Which of the following statements is true?

(A) The most common presentation of primary hyperparathyroidism is asymptomatic hypercalcemia

(B) A positive family history indicates chief cell hyperplasia

(C) Renal complications from primary hyperparathyroidism are becoming increasingly uncommon

(D) In the absence of renal failure, serum phosphate should be low

(E) All of the above

250. A regularly seen 37-year-old is suspected of being a lesbian. True statements about lesbians include that

(A) a small minority of lesbians would like to have children

(B) their behavior is due to an abnormal hormonal state

(C) they have been found to have different personality characteristics from other women

(D) the great majority of lesbians are quite open in telling their physicians about their lesbianism

(E) lesbians who do not inform their physicians of their situation refrain out of fear of jeopardizing their medical care

251. A 44-year-old patient is found to have increased venous pressure with edema of the upper body, cyanosis, dilated subcutaneous collateral vessels in the chest, and headache. He is diagnosed with superior vena cava syndrome. What is the most likely underlying condition in this patient?

(A) Bronchogenic carcinoma
(B) Constrictive pericarditis
(C) Histoplasmosis (sclerosing mediastinitis)
(D) Substernal thyroid
(E) Thoracic aortic aneurysm

252. A 7-year-old girl is referred for evaluation of vaginal bleeding for 2 months. The mother says that she has not been exposed to exogenous estrogens. Physical examination reveals height at the 98th percentile, Tanner stage III breast development, and no axillary or pubic hair. No abdominal or pelvic masses are palpated. Neurologic examination is normal. Radiographic and laboratory evaluations reveal the following:

Skull films: normal sella; no intracerebral calcifications
Bone age: 10 years
Urinary 17-ketosteroids: 1.7 μmol (0.5 mg)/g creatinine/24 h
Urinary gonadotropins: undetectable

The appropriate next step in the management of this girl would be

(A) abdominal CT scanning and pelvic sonography
(B) exploratory laparotomy
(C) karyotype analysis
(D) measurement of plasma androstenedione level
(E) treatment with medroxyprogesterone acetate

253. A 32-year-old non-smoking black female has been under a colleague's care for one year. She initially presented with dyspnea, cough, and nodular skin lesions. These symptoms resolved with colchicine. She presents now with acute right flank pain and hematuria. The most likely diagnosis is

(A) pre-existing sarcoidosis with development of renal infarction
(B) pre-existing Wegener's granulomatosis with glomerulonephritis
(C) pre-existing sarcoidosis with urinary tract calculi and obstruction
(D) primary pulmonary hypertension with renal vein thrombosis
(E) reactive airways disease with pyelonephritis

254. A 50-year-old male presents with a history of hypertension and flank pain. His father died of renal failure at age 60 and an uncle and brother both died of cerebral hemorrhage in their forties. The patient's serum creatinine is moderately elevated. An ultrasound of the abdomen is obtained and reveals bilateral renal cysts in enlarged kidneys. Which of the following statements is true?

(A) Children of the patient are not likely to develop renal cysts
(B) Progressive renal failure should be anticipated
(C) Cyst aspiration is desirable to confirm the diagnosis and treat the hypertension
(D) Cerebral angiography is warranted to rule out aneurysm
(E) Fluid restriction should be instituted

255. A 67-year-old woman, who has previously been healthy, undergoes emergency surgery for a ruptured abdominal aortic aneurysm. Intraoperatively, she requires 8 units of packed red blood cells to maintain her blood pressure and hematocrit. Following surgery she is hemodynamically stable. On the third postoperative day she appears jaundiced, but abdominal examination is unremarkable and she is afebrile. Total serum bilirubin concentration at this time is 141 μmol/L (8.3 mg/dL) (direct, 107 μmol/L [6.3 mg/dL]). Serum alkaline phosphatase level is 110 units, and serum AST level is 0.85 μkat/L (51 Karmen units/mL). The most likely explanation for the woman's jaundice is

(A) a stone in the common bile duct

(B) acute hepatic infarct

(C) benign intrahepatic cholestasis

(D) halothane hepatitis

(E) posttransfusion hepatitis

256. Which of the following clinical features is most typically associated with a Pancoast's tumor?

(A) Atelectasis of the adjacent apical lung segment

(B) Horner's syndrome

(C) Nonproductive cough

(D) Absence of pain

257. At 25 weeks of gestation, an amniocentesis is performed on an Rh-isoimmunized patient with an anti-D titer of 1:126 and a nonhydropic fetus. The OD_{450} result of 0.26 is placed high in zone II on the Liley scale. You should now

(A) determine the spouse's blood type

(B) repeat the maternal serum antibody titer

(C) repeat the ultrasound examination and amniocentesis

(D) perform an immediate intrauterine transfusion

(E) prepare for termination of pregnancy

258. A 62-year-old woman has been taking quinidine sulfate because of asymptomatic ventricular couplets. One week later, she was admitted to the hospital after a syncopal episode. Serum electrolyte concentrations were normal. The arrhythmia shown below appeared transiently on her cardiac monitor.

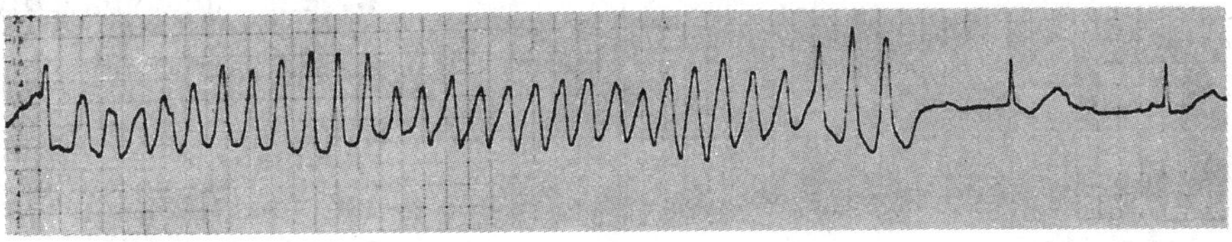

The recommended course at this time is to

(A) increase the quinidine dose

(B) discontinue administration of quinidine and observe

(C) begin intravenous administration of procainamide 2 mg/min

(D) administer sodium bicarbonate, 70 meq, intravenously

(E) administer potassium chloride, 10 meq, intravenously over 1 h

Questions 259-260: A 58-year-old smoker with emphysema notes increased sputum production for four days. He is brought to an emergency room after his wife called the ambulance when he became suddenly short of breath and confused. He is given oxygen by mask by the ambulance crew. On arrival at the hospital he is somnolent. He has marked peripheral edema and ascites. His hemoglobin is 180 g/L (18 g/dL) and arterial blood gases are pH 7.08, P_{O_2} 148 mmHg, and P_{CO_2} 106 mmHg.

259. The most appropriate immediate therapy for the man described above would be

(A) administration of isoetharine by air-compressor nebulizer

(B) discontinuation of supplemental oxygen

(C) endotracheal intubation and assisted ventilation

(D) intravenous infusion of sodium bicarbonate

(E) subcutaneous injection of epinephrine

260. For the patient described above, right ventricular heart failure would be treated with

(A) diazoxide

(B) digoxin

(C) hydralazine

(D) oxygen

(E) phlebotomy

261. A 35-year-old former hemodialysis nurse is seen because of a 6-month history of fatigue and amenorrhea. On examination she has a scleral icterus, a mildly tender liver, and a tibial rash consistent with erythema nodosum. ALT and AST levels are both in the range of 1.5 μkat/L (100 U/L) and bilirubin is 51.3 μmol/L (3 mg/dL), while alkaline phosphatase and serum albumin levels are normal. Hepatitis serology detects HBsAg and IgG anti-HBcAg. Liver biopsy discloses a mononuclear cell portal infiltrate and hepatocyte destruction at the periphery of the lobules. Which of the following therapeutic strategies is best?

(A) Administration of low-dose cyclophosphamide, 50 mg/d for 2 months

(B) Administration of prednisone, 20 to 40 mg/d for 2 months and then taper-based on response

(C) Administration of prednisone, 10 mg every other day for 3 months

(D) Administration of acyclovir, 400 mg every 6 h for 2 weeks

(E) Referral to a medical center participating in a trial of alpha interferon

262. Which of the following statements is true regarding scleroderma?

(A) Gastrointestinal manifestations include esophageal dysmotility and wide-mouth colonic diverticula

(B) Pseudoobstruction is uncommon

(C) Pneumatosis intestinalis is an ominous finding when associated with scleroderma

(D) Malabsorption seldom results from small bowel hypomotility

(E) GI manifestations in the absence of cutaneous manifestations should preclude the diagnosis of scleroderma

263. A patient with endometriosis undergoes total abdominal hysterectomy and bilateral salpingo-oophorectomy. Findings at surgery include a 7-cm right-sided endometrioma and uterosacral nodularity. Hemorrhage makes exposure difficult. On postoperative day 2, the patient develops a temperature of 38.2°C (100.8°F), and on postoperative day 4, begins to complain of right flank pain. The most likely diagnosis is

(A) appendicitis

(B) cecal rupture

(C) pelvic cellulitis

(D) right ureteral ligation

(E) perinephric abscess

264. A 50-year-old man with a history of organomegaly and an elevated hematocrit without apparent secondary cause was well until the sudden onset of right upper quadrant pain. On examination the patient is afebrile and has clear lungs, normal cardiac function, an abdominal fluid wave, splenomegaly, and a markedly enlarged liver with a palpable, very tender edge. Liver function tests are normal except for mild elevation of hepatic transaminases. Which of the following is the most appropriate procedure for purposes of establishing a diagnosis?

(A) Abdominal ultrasound

(B) CT scan of the liver

(C) Hepatic venography

(D) Paracentesis

(E) Radionuclide liver-spleen scan

265. A 42-year-old woman presents with a complaint of watery diarrhea that has occurred intermittently over the past 4 years. After the passage of three or four loose stools in the morning, she feels well for the rest of the day and never has nocturnal diarrhea. Physical examination reveals an anxious woman with a tender left lower abdominal quadrant and no fecal material in the rectum; the results are otherwise normal. Sigmoidoscopic examination discloses excess mucus, but the mucosa appears normal. Barium enema is normal except for sigmoid spasticity, and examination of a stool specimen reveals well-formed feces that are negative for blood, pathogenic bacteria, and parasites. Results of thyroid studies are normal. A trial of milk restriction results in no change in symptoms. She is concerned her symptoms are "psychologic." At this point the physician should

(A) consider a trial of diphenoxylate or paregoric to control symptomatic diarrhea

(B) tell the patient that her symptoms are largely emotional in origin

(C) consider a trial of psyllium to increase stool bulk

(D) obtain stool electrolytes and osmolality

(E) perform a jejunal aspirate and analyze the fluid for parasites

266. Which of the following characteristics is true regarding hepatitis A?

(A) Urogenital mode of transmission

(B) Insidious onset

(C) High malignancy potential

(D) Prognosis is better than in hepatitis B and C

(E) Carrier state in up to 50 percent of affected patients

267. Following an appendectomy for acute appendicitis, a 1.5-cm carcinoid tumor was detected in the appendectomy specimens. Which of the following statements is true for this tumor?

(A) The patient should be advised to undergo ileocolectomy

(B) The most common location of carcinoids is in the appendix

(C) The carcinoid syndrome occurs in more than half the patients with carcinoid tumors

(D) The tumor is an apudoma

(E) Patients with carcinoid tumors often suffer from diarrhea

268. A patient with ovarian carcinoma is referred to your office. What most likely are her presenting symptoms?

(A) Abdominal distention and pain

(B) Constipation and frequent urination

(C) Nausea and vaginal discharge

(D) Vaginal bleeding and anorexia

(E) Weight loss and dyspareunia

269. A 37-year-old man with chronic alcoholism is admitted to the hospital with acute pancreatitis. On the third hospital day, sudden, complete blindness develops in the left eye. The most likely explanation is

(A) acute glaucoma

(B) alcohol withdrawal symptoms

(C) occlusion of the retinal vein

(D) Purtscher's retinopathy

(E) transient ischemic attack (transient monocular blindness)

270. A 35-year-old patient in good health undergoes a hysterectomy for CIS of the cervix. Postoperatively, she is administered 5% dextrose and 0.45% NaCl at 150 mL/h. On the fourth postoperative day, the patient inadvertently has serum electrolytes drawn; the nurse calls to inquire about filing an incident report and also gives you the test results: Na^+ 129, K^+ 3.1, Cl^- 100, CO_2 22. Urinary output is brisk. You should

(A) correct the sodium deficit with hypertonic saline and add KCl to the IV

(B) draw stat urine electrolytes and serum BUN/creatinine to determine optimal IV fluid management

(C) decrease the IV rate and add KCl to the IV

(D) correct the sodium deficit with normal saline and add KCl to the IV

(E) chastise the nurse for not paying close attention to your orders and inform her that the electrolytes are in the acceptable range for the fourth postoperative day

271. During a regular physical examination, it is observed that a 2-year-old asymptomatic patient has a systolic murmur, hypertension, and diminished femoral pulses. Which of the following statements about this child's disorder is correct?

(A) Claudication is frequently noted

(B) Corrective surgery has a greater than 5 percent mortality

(C) Immediate surgery is indicated

(D) Rib notching is often seen on x-ray

(E) The life expectancy without surgery is only a few years

272. A 64-year-old man with insulin-dependent adult-onset diabetes mellitus seeks emergency medical treament after 2 days of increasingly severe abdominal pain of the right upper quadrant, which has spread over the entire abdomen and is associated with nausea, vomiting, fever, and chills. On examination, he is alert and oriented but appears to be quite acutely distressed. Vital signs are temperature, 39.4°C (103°F); pulse, 140 beats per minute; and blood pressure, 100/60 mmHg. His sclerae are mildly icteric. His abdomen is diffusely tender with marked guarding in the right upper quadrant; there is no palpable hepatosplenomegaly, and there are no audible bowel sounds. Rectal examination reveals no focal tenderness; stool is guaiac-negative. Laboratory values are as follows:

Hematocrit: 34 percent

White blood cell count: 22,500/mm^3 with a marked left shift

Plasma glucose: 17.8 mmol/L (325 mg/dL)

Blood urea nitrogen: 10.5 μmol/L (30 mg/dL)

Serum AST: 2.1 μkat/L (125 Karmen units/mL)

Serum alkaline phosphatase: 210 units

Serum amylase: 3.3 μkat/L (200 U/dL)

His abdominal flat-plate x-ray is shown below.

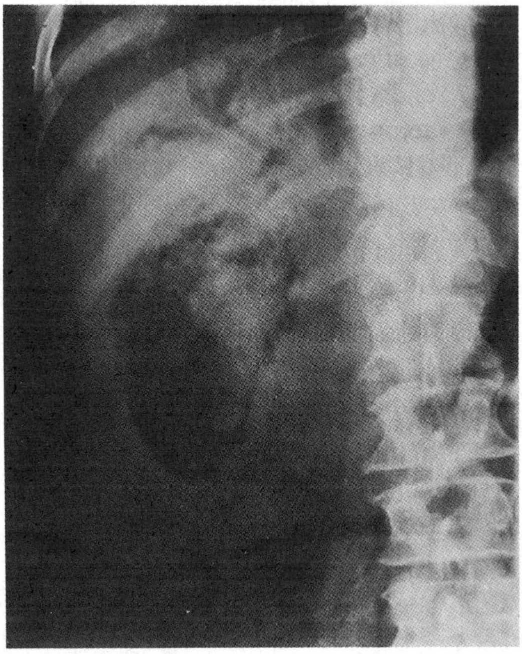

The most appropriate management at this point would be to order

(A) conservative medical measures only for the next 48 to 72 h

(B) an abdominal ultrasound examination

(C) an upper gastrointestinal examination with Gastrografin dye

(D) endoscopic retrograde cholangiopancreatography

(E) preparations for an emergency laparotomy

273. A 17-year-old presents to the emergency room with right lower quadrant pain, fever, and leukocytosis. Surgical consultation confirms your clinical impression of acute appendicitis. At surgery, the appendix is normal. What is the most common condition likely to be found at surgery?

(A) Acute gastroenteritis

(B) Mesenteric lymphadenitis

(C) No organic disease

(D) Pelvic inflammatory disease

(E) Ruptured ovarian cyst

274. Administration of which of the following drugs or classes of drugs has been shown to prolong survival in persons with acute pancreatitis?

(A) Antibiotics

(B) Anticholinergics

(C) Aprotinin (Trasylol)

(D) Cimetidine

(E) None of the above

275. True statements about ovarian neoplasms in children include which of the following?

(A) They are most often of germ cell origin

(B) They are an infrequent cause of precocious puberty

(C) Coelomic epithelial tumors are usually benign

(D) Tumors of germ cell origin are frequently malignant

(E) All of the above

276. A 48-year-old patient has invasive cervical carcinoma. Which of the following statements best describes her disease?

(A) Early symptoms include watery, blood-tinged vaginal discharge and postcoital spotting

(B) Involvement of periaortic lymph nodes is present in up to 20 percent of stage I tumors

(C) For early-stage disease (I and IIA), survival is better with radical surgery compared with radiation therapy

(D) Recurrent carcinoma is very sensitive to chemotherapy

(E) Intraarterial chemotherapy has had a major impact on survival

277. Which of the following statements regarding diverticular disease of the colon is true?

(A) The diverticulum involves all layers of the colonic wall

(B) Most cases of diverticulitis result in peridiverticular inflammation secondary to mechanical factors which compromise the vascular supply of the diverticula

(C) Acute diverticulitis usually requires surgical excision

(D) Hematochezia in elderly patients seldom results from hemorrhage due to diverticula

(E) Right-sided diverticula are of little significance because of the liquid composition of stool in the proximal colon

278. Which of the following statements concerning bronchial carcinoid tumors is true?

(A) They frequently metastasize

(B) They most commonly arise in the major proximal bronchi

(C) They produce the carcinoid syndrome

(D) They are radiosensitive

(E) They result in a relatively short-term survival rate

279. Which of the following statements best characterizes the hemolysis associated with glucose 6-phosphate dehydrogenase (G6PD) deficiency?

(A) It is more severe in affected blacks than in affected persons of Mediterranean ancestry

(B) It is more severe in females than in males

(C) It causes the appearance of Heinz bodies on Wright staining of a peripheral smear

(D) It most often is precipitated by infection

(E) The best time to perform the diagnostic test is during a hemolytic crisis

280. Estrogen replacement therapy, ERT, has been shown to

(A) increase the risk of developing breast and ovarian cancer

(B) provide protection against atherosclerotic coronary heart disease

(C) increase levels of low-density lipoprotein

(D) increase the risk of developing osteoporosis

281. A 48-year-old man is admitted to the coronary care unit with an acute inferior myocardial infarction. Two hours after admission, his blood pressure is 86/52 mmHg; his heart rate is 40 beats per minute with sinus rhythm. Which of the following would be the most appropriate initial therapy?

(A) Immediate insertion of a temporary transvenous pacemaker

(B) Intravenous administration of atropine sulfate, 0.6 mg

(C) Administration of normal saline, 300 mL over 15 min

(D) Intravenous administration of dobutamine, 0.35 mg/min

(E) Intravenous administration of isoproterenol, 5.0 μg/min

282. To determine whether a child with paroxysmal coughing and gasping has whooping cough, a physician would do best to order

(A) blood cultures

(B) chest x-ray

(C) Gram stain of the sputum

(D) lateral x-ray of the neck

(E) white blood cell count and differential

283. Progestin and estrogen-containing birth control pills achieve their contraceptive effect by

(A) inhibition of ovulation

(B) improved penetrability of sperm into the cervical mucus

(C) hypertrophic changes of the endometrium impairing implantation

(D) uterotubal hypermotility impairing sperm transport

284. A 20-year-old man was found to have ulcerative proctitis 2 years ago. Mild rectal bleeding was well controlled on daily steroid enemas, which were discontinued a year ago. For the last 3 months, he has had increasingly frequent bloody diarrhea (now 6 to 10 times a day), lower abdominal cramps, low-grade fever, anorexia, and a 5-kg (11-lb) weight loss. Physical examination of this thin, pale young man, who appears acutely ill, reveals these vital signs: temperature, 37.8°C (100°F); pulse, 110 beats per minute; and blood pressure, 120/70 mmHg. The lower abdomen is mildly and diffusely tender, but there is no rebound tenderness and bowel sounds are active. Stool is grossly bloody. Sigmoidoscopy, limited to 10 cm because of discomfort, shows marked mucosal erythema and friability; diffuse ulceration is present, and an exudate contains pus and blood.

Three hours after a barium enema, which shows ulcerations throughout the colon, the man's abdominal pain markedly worsens. Vital signs now are temperature, 39.6°C (103.2°F); pulse, 130 beats per minute; and blood pressure, 90/60 mmHg. On examination the abdomen is distended and diffusely tender with rebound; bowel sounds are infrequent. An abdominal flat-plate x-ray is pictured below.

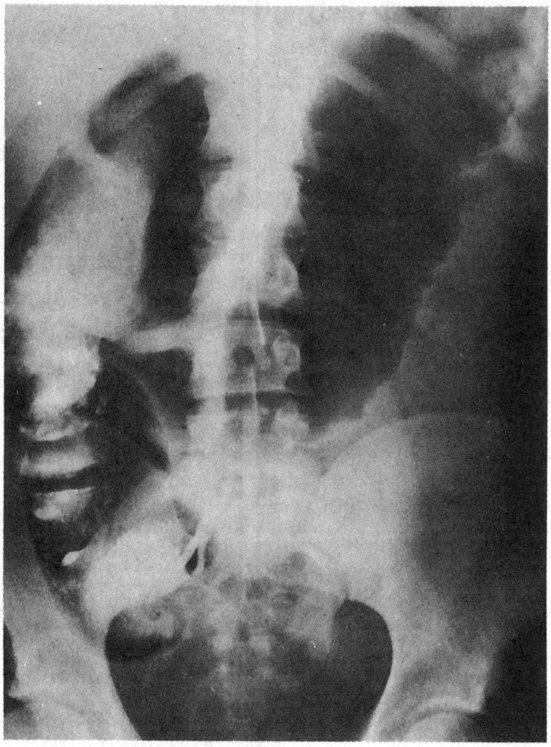

The most likely diagnosis for the disorder described above is

(A) acute colonic perforation

(B) inferior mesenteric artery occlusion

(C) nonthrombic mesenteric ischemia

(D) toxic megacolon

(E) volvulus

285. A previously healthy 58-year-old man is admitted to the hospital because of an acute inferior myocardial infarction. Within several hours, he becomes oliguric and hypotensive (blood pressure is 90/60 mmHg). Insertion of a pulmonary artery (Swan-Ganz) catheter reveals the following pressures: pulmonary capillary wedge, 4 mmHg; pulmonary artery, 22/4 mmHg; and mean right atrial, 11 mmHg. This man would best be treated with

(A) digoxin

(B) dopamine

(C) fluids

(D) intraaortic balloon counterpulsation

(E) norepinephrine

286. Which of the following statements regarding pulmonary thromboembolism is true?

(A) It is associated with clinically apparent deep vein thrombosis in more than 50 percent of patients

(B) It induces a reflex, possibly serotonin-mediated bronchoconstriction

(C) It rarely causes hypoxemia owing to only a slight ventilation-perfusion imbalance

(D) It must occlude less than 10 percent of the pulmonary vascular bed to produce symptoms in a previously healthy patient

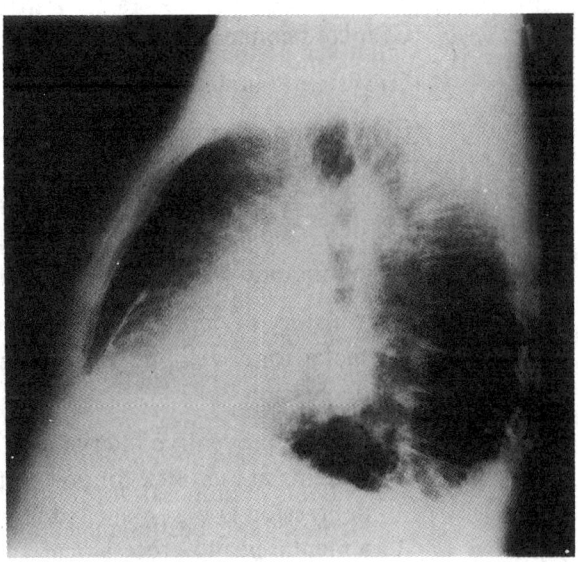

287. Which of the following physical findings is associated with the chest x-ray shown above?

(A) Central cyanosis

(B) Late-peaking systolic ejection murmur

(C) Opening snap and diastolic rumble

(D) Pericardial knock

(E) Wide splitting of the second heart sound

288. For the last 2 years, a 27-year-old man has had recurrent episodes of asymmetrical inflammatory oligoarticular arthritis involving his knees, ankles, and elbows lasting from 2 to 4 weeks. He also states he has had recurrent, painful "canker sores" in his mouth for the last 10 years. Now, he presents with fever, arthritis, mild abdominal pain, severe headache, and superficial thrombophlebitis in the left leg. The most likely diagnosis in this man is

(A) Behçet's syndrome
(B) regional enteritis
(C) systemic lupus erythematosus
(D) ulcerative colitis
(E) Whipple's disease

289. A 15-year-old boy presents to the emergency room with acute testicular pain of 4 h duration. He is noted to have a high-riding, indurated, and markedly tender left testis. Urinalysis is unremarkable. Correct statements regarding the patient include which of the following?

(A) There is a strong likelihood that this patient's father or brother has had or will have a similar event
(B) Surgery should be delayed until a technetium scan clarifies the diagnosis
(C) The majority of testicles that have undergone torsion can be salvaged if surgery is performed within 24 h
(D) If torsion is found, both testes should undergo orchiopexy
(E) The patient is likely to have a positive Prehn's sign

290. A 37-year-old woman with Raynaud's phenomenon complains of progressive weakness with inability to arise out of a sitting position without assistance. On examination, the patient has swollen "sausage-like" fingers, alopecia, erythematous patches on the knuckles, facial telangiectasias, and proximal muscle weakness. Laboratory evaluation includes a normal CBC and serum chemistries, except for creatine phosphokinase 4.5 μkat/L (270 U/L) and aldolase 500 nkat/L (30 U/L). The following serologic profile is found: rheumatoid factor is positive at 1:1600; ANA is also positive at 1:1600 with a speckled pattern and very high titers of antibodies against the ribonuclease-sensitive ribonucleoprotein component of extractable nuclear antigen. This patient probably has

(A) dermatomyositis
(B) early rheumatoid arthritis
(C) mixed connective tissue disease
(D) systemic lupus erythematosus
(E) systemic sclerosis

291. True statements regarding postpartum depression include which of the following?

(A) A history of depression is not a risk factor for developing postpartum depression
(B) Prenatal preventive intervention for patients at high risk for postpartum depression is best managed alone by a mental health professional
(C) Postpartum depression is a self-limiting process that lasts for a maximum of 3 months
(D) About 10 to 12 percent of women develop postpartum depression

292. A 25-year-old man has had pain and swelling in the right knee for the last year. He is otherwise well and gives no history of trauma. X-rays show several erosions at the margin of the right knee joint. Aspiration of the joint yields 25 mL of dark-brown synovial fluid. The most likely diagnosis is

(A) atypical rheumatoid arthritis

(B) hemangioma

(C) incomplete Reiter's syndrome

(D) osteochondritis dissecans

(E) pigmented villonodular synovitis

293. Upon biopsy, seminoma is diagnosed in a 59-year-old patient. Seminoma is accurately described by which of the following statements?

(A) It is a rare type of testicular cancer

(B) Metastases to liver and bone are frequently found

(C) It is a very radiosensitive tumor

(D) The 5-year survival rate approaches 50 percent

(E) It is a rapidly growing tumor

294. Which of the following statements regarding Reiter's syndrome is true?

(A) It follows an enteric infection

(B) It is highly associated with histocompatibility antigen HLA-B27

(C) Enthesitis often occurs at the Achilles tendon and plantar fascia insertion sites

(D) Venerally-acquired reactive arthritis is predominantly a male disease

(E) All of the above are true

295. A 25-year-old, previously healthy woman presents with jaundice, confusion, and fever. Initial physical examination is unremarkable except for scattered petechiae on the lower extremities, scleral icterus, and disorientation on mental status examination. Laboratory examination discloses the following: hematocrit, 27 percent; white cell count, 12,000/μL; platelet count, 10,000/μL; bilirubin, 85 μmol/L (5 mg/dL); direct bilirubin, 10 μmol/L (0.6 mg/dL); urea nitrogen, 21 mmol/L (60 mg/dL); creatinine, 400 μmol/L (4.5 mg/dL). Red blood cell smear discloses fragmented red blood cells and nucleated red blood cells. Prothrombin, thrombin, and partial thromboplastin times are all normal. The most effective and appropriate therapeutic maneuver is likely to be

(A) administration of aspirin

(B) administration of high-dose glucocorticoids

(C) administration of high-dose glucocorticoids plus cyclophosphamide

(D) plasmapheresis

(E) splenectomy

296. A 38-year-old white male presents with sinus pain and bloody discharge. Nasal exam shows nasal ulcerations. Which of the following findings supports the diagnosis of Wegener's granulomatosis?

(A) Cavitary pulmonary lesion

(B) Well-defined multinucleated giant cells within the pulmonary granulomas

(C) Relentless progression from proteinuria to renal failure

(D) Negative antineutrophil cytoplasmic antibody

(E) Treatment with cyclophosphamide is ineffective and avoided due to bone marrow suppression

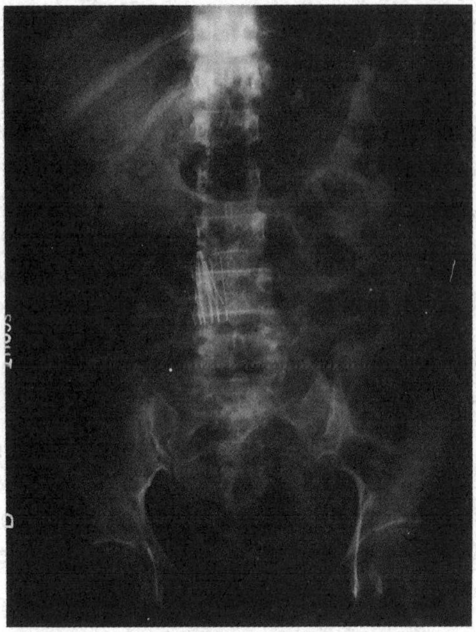

297. Indications for placement of the device pictured in the abdominal x-ray shown above include

(A) recurrent pulmonary embolus despite adequate anticoagulation therapy

(B) axillary vein thrombosis

(C) a single pulmonary embolus

(D) pulmonary embolus due to deep vein thrombosis of the lower extremity occurring 2 weeks postoperatively

---

298. A 72-year-old man who has become progressively fatigued is found to be anemic. Hematologic laboratory values are as follows:

Hemoglobin: 100 g/L (10 g/dL)
Hematocrit: 27.5 percent
Mean corpuscular volume (MCV): 101 fL
Mean corpuscular hemoglobin (MCH): 30 pg
Mean corpuscular hemoglobin concentration (MCHC): 340 g/L (34 g/dL)
Reticulocyte count: 0.5 percent
White blood cell count: 7300/mm^3 (65 percent neutrophils)
Platelet count: 210,000/mm^3

The most likely diagnosis is

(A) acute leukemia

(B) aplastic anemia

(C) autoimmune hemolytic anemia

(D) iron-deficiency

(E) myelodysplastic syndrome

299. Which of the following statements regarding schwannomas is true?

(A) They are central nerve tumors

(B) The vestibulocochlear nerve is often affected

(C) They arise most frequently in motor nerves

(D) They often degenerate to malignancy

(E) They represent nearly 75 percent of all intracranial neoplasms

300. A 38-year-old father of four is scheduled for a vasectomy. It is explained to him that it is a highly reliable form of birth control but not without some risk. Vasectomy has been associated with which of the following complications?

(A) Hematoma

(B) Infection

(C) Sperm granulomas

(D) Spontaneous reanastomosis

(E) All of the above

301. A neurological referral has confirmed a diagnosis of craniopharyngioma in your patient. Which of the following statements concerning these tumors is correct?

(A) They originate from mesoderm and are rarely cystic

(B) They are nearly always malignant with a poor prognosis

(C) They may cause compression of optic tracts and visual symptoms

(D) They most commonly appear in adults after the fifth decade

302. A 21-year-old woman who has had severe menorrhagia is referred by her gynecologist for evaluation of a possible systemic coagulopathy. A younger sister has been noted to bleed excessively after trauma. She takes no medications; physical examination is unremarkable. Initial laboratory results include the following: platelet count, 252,000/mm^3; prothrombin time, 23.6 s (control 11.6 s); and partial thromboplastin time, 26.9 s (control 33.3 s). Further laboratory testing should consist of

(A) determination of alpha$_2$-antiplasmin level

(B) determination of bleeding time

(C) determination of factor VII level

(D) determination of factor VIII level

(E) screening for inhibitors

303. Which of the following statements concerning the prognosis of pernicious anemia is true?

(A) The presence of antiparietal-cell antibodies is diagnostic of pernicious anemia

(B) Hematologic response to folate therapy alone rules out pernicious anemia as the cause of megaloblastic anemia

(C) Hyperkalemia may be a consequence of vitamin B_{12} therapy

(D) Bone marrow examination would be expected to reveal marked depletion of erythrocyte precursors in persons with untreated pernicious anemia

(E) Serum gastrin levels usually are elevated in persons with pernicious anemia

304. A 27-year-old woman has habitual abortion from luteal insufficiency. Which of the following regimens of progesterone therapy is appropriate in the luteal phase of the menstrual cycle in this case?

(A) Progesterone vaginal suppository, 25 mg twice daily

(B) Progesterone vaginal suppository, 50 mg twice daily

(C) Progesterone in oil, 12.5 mg IM weekly

(D) Hydroxyprogesterone caproate, 250 mg IM weekly

(E) Medroxyprogesterone acetate, 100 mg IM weekly

305. A 14-year-old boy has a history of recurrent respiratory infections with *Staphylococcus aureus* and *Aspergillus fumigatus*. When he was 7 years old he had a hepatic abscess that was drained surgically; no organism was cultured, but the problem responded to drainage and prolonged antibiotic therapy. His parents and two younger siblings are healthy, but an older brother died in infancy of infection. The laboratory study most likely to assist in establishing the diagnosis is

(A) determination of leukocyte myeloperoxidase level

(B) quantitative determination of serum immunoglobulin levels

(C) T-lymphocyte functional and subpopulation assessment

(D) nitroblue tetrazolium reduction test

(E) bone marrow aspiration and biopsy

306. Maternal diabetes mellitus is associated with which of the following symptoms in the fetus or neonate?

(A) Delayed pulmonic maturity in the fetus

(B) Hypocalcemia in the newborn

(C) Hypoglycemia in the newborn

(D) Macrosomia in the fetus

(E) All of the above

307. A 19-year-old student has dysuria and a vaginal discharge. She is noted to have a bilateral groin rash, vaginal erythema, and a chunky white vaginal discharge. The laboratory test most likely to detect a specific host-defense defect causing this clinical problem would be

(A) blood glucose concentration

(B) blood urea nitrogen concentration

(C) serum immunoglobulin A concentration

(D) serum immunoglobulin E concentration

(E) serum complement concentration

308. The best way to establish the diagnosis of cryptosporidiosis in a patient with AIDS and watery diarrhea is

(A) acid-fast staining of concentrated stool

(B) acute and convalescent serologic studies

(C) Gram stain of stool

(D) stool culture

(E) wet mount of stool

309. A posterolateral herniation at the interspace between L4 and L5 may produce

(A) exaggeration of dorsiflexion of the great toe

(B) sensory deficit on the lateral aspect of the foot

(C) hyperesthesia on the dorsum of the foot

(D) weakness on plantar flexion

310. Which of the following organisms often causes diarrhea, confusion, and delirium in conjunction with pneumonia?

(A) *Francisella tularensis*

(B) *Haemophilus pneumoniae*

(C) *Klebsiella pneumoniae*

(D) *Legionella pneumophila*

(E) *Mycoplasma pneumoniae*

311. There are approximately 400 to 700 minor salivary glands in the oral cavity. Pleomorphic adenomas (mixed tumors) can occur in any of them and are characterized by which of the following?

(A) They are irregularly shaped tumors

(B) They are rapid-growing

(C) They tend to recur if simply enucleated

(D) They present as rock-hard masses

312. *Listeria monocytogenes* most frequently causes which of the following infections?

(A) Conjunctivitis

(B) Endocarditis

(C) Hepatitis

(D) Meningitis

(E) Peritonitis

---

313. At the time of delivery, a woman is noted to have a large volume of amniotic fluid. At 6 h of age her baby begins regurgitating small amounts of mucus and bile-stained fluid. Physical examination of the infant is normal, and an abdominal x-ray is obtained (shown).

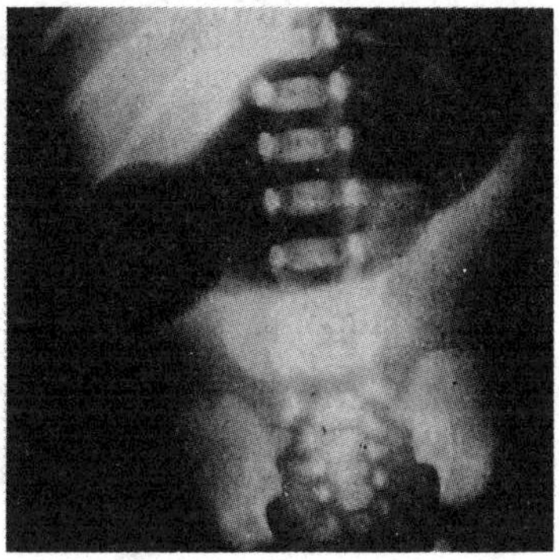

The most likely diagnosis of this infant's disorder is

(A) duodenal atresia

(B) esophageal atresia

(C) gastric duplication

(D) midgut volvulus

(E) pyloric stenosis

314. Which of the following pleural-fluid samples is most suggestive of tuberculous pleuritis?

Fluid sample	Color	pH	Protein, g/L	Glucose, mmol/L	LDH, U/mL	WBC Total (per mm³)	WBC % Lymphocytes
(A)	Clear yellow	7.15	35	1.1	600	2,000	95
(B)	Thick green	7.00	40	1.1	600	10,000	50
(C)	Clear yellow	7.30	15	4.4	150	200	50
(D)	Pink-tinged	7.40	30	4.4	600	3,000	50
(E)	Clear yellow	7.30	35	3.3	150	2,000	95

(LDH, lactate dehydrogenase; WBC, white blood cell count)

Questions 315-316: An 18-year-old sexually active woman presents to the emergency room with fever and right upper quadrant and lower abdominal pain. She has mucopurulent cervicitis and tenderness with cervical motion. The right upper quadrant, uterine fundus, and adnexa are slightly tender.

315. Which of the following agents is the most likely cause of this clinical syndrome?

(A) *Chlamydia trachomatis*

(B) Herpes simplex

(C) *Mycoplasma hominis*

(D) *Neisseria gonorrhoeae*

(E) Syphilis

316. Laboratory studies and ultrasound of the pelvis and right lower quadrant exclude pregnancy and appendicitis. Which of the following antibiotic regimens is the best choice?

(A) Acyclovir plus penicillin

(B) Doxycycline alone

(C) Doxycycline plus cefoxitin

(D) Metronidazole plus gentamicin

(E) Penicillin alone

Questions 317-318: A hospital employee rushes to the emergency room 10 minutes after accidentally getting splashed in the eye with bleach. He is agitated and in pain.

317. The emergency room physician should first

(A) measure the patient's visual acuity

(B) instill a topical antibiotic eyedrop

(C) irrigate the eye copiously with saline

(D) sedate the patient to ease examination and treatment

(E) examine the other eye

318. Which of the following is the most urgent eye emergency?

(A) Retinal detachment

(B) Vitreous hemorrhage

(C) Glaucoma

(D) Central retinal artery occlusion

(E) Perforation of the eyeball

319. The subclavian steal syndrome is associated with which of the following hemodynamic abnormalities?

(A) Occlusion of a vertebral artery

(B) Occlusion of the subclavian artery

(C) Venous occlusive disease

(D) Upper extremity venous congestion

320. Prognosis in ovarian serous cystadenocarcinoma is influenced by

(A) extent of the tumor

(B) volume of the tumor

(C) histologic differentiation of the tumor

(D) presence of ascites

(E) all of the above

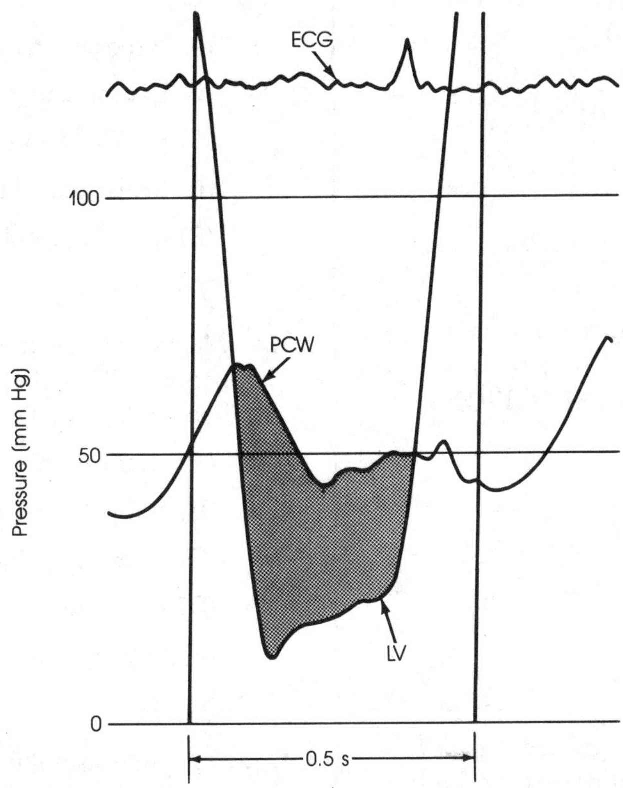

From Grossman W (ed): *Cardiac Catheterization and Angiography*, 3d ed. Philadelphia, Lea & Febiger, 1986, with permission.

321. The figure above most likely represents the pulmonary capillary wedge and left ventricular pressure tracing from which of the following patients?

(A) A 40-year-old woman with a history of rheumatic fever, orthopnea, and hemoptysis

(B) A 24-year-old intravenous drug abuser with fever, holosystolic murmur, and large mitral valve vegetation

(C) A 26-year-old man with long arms, abnormal lenses, and a diastolic murmur

(D) A 72-year-old man with left ventricular hypertrophy, syncope, and a systolic murmur

(E) A 35-year-old woman with elevated neck veins and a large mediastinal mass due to non-Hodgkin's lymphoma

DIRECTIONS (Questions 322-324): Each question below contains four or five suggested responses. Select the **EXACT** number of responses indicated by each question.

322. A group of congenital anomalies known collectively as Potter syndrome includes renal agenesis (or other renal anomalies) and pulmonary hypoplasia. Other anomalies associated with Potter syndrome include **(SELECT 2 CHOICES)**

(A) amnion nodosum

(B) cleft palate

(C) hydrocephaly

(D) oligohydramnios

323. Which of the following maternal infections are associated with fetal congenital anomalies? **(SELECT 2 INFECTIONS)**

(A) Common cold

(B) Cytomegalovirus

(C) Influenza

(D) Mumps

(E) Rubella

324. A 27-year-old woman, gravida 2, para 1, with an otherwise normal pregnancy complains of decreased fetal movement at 38 weeks' gestation. Appropriate management options would include which of the following?
(SELECT 3 MANAGEMENT OPTIONS)

(A) Amniocentesis

(B) Biophysical profile (BPP)

(C) Contraction stress test (CST)

(D) Immediate delivery

(E) Nonstress test (NST)

DIRECTIONS (Questions 325-346): Each **NEGATIVELY** phrased question below contains four or five suggested responses. Select the **one best** response to each question.

325. A patient is diagnosed with cancer of the urinary bladder. Which of the following factors in the patient's history probably is NOT associated with carcinoma of the bladder?

(A) Exposure to cigarette smoke

(B) Exposure to dyes

(C) Positive family history

(D) Schistosomal infestation

(E) Use of cyclophosphamide

326. Magnetic resonance imaging (MRI) is superior to CT in the evaluation of all the following EXCEPT

(A) arteriovenous malformation

(B) multiple sclerosis

(C) subarachnoid hemorrhage

(D) syringomyelia

(E) vertebral osteomyelitis

327. Digoxin is useful in the treatment of congestive heart failure. Which of the following factors would NOT be expected to contribute to digitalis toxicity?

(A) Addition of quinidine to the therapeutic regimen

(B) Chronic obstructive lung disease with hypoxemia

(C) Diuretic therapy with loop diuretics

(D) Hyperparathyroidism

(E) Hyperthyroidism

328. All the following are risk factors for development of cancer of the colon EXCEPT

(A) adenomatous polyps

(B) Crohn's colitis

(C) juvenile polyposis

(D) ulcerative colitis

(E) uterosigmoidostomy

329. A 52-year-old white female presents with fatigue. Her routine screening laboratory values reveal a three-fold increase in the alkaline phosphatase level. Serum bilirubin is normal. Which of the following features is NOT consistent with the diagnosis of primary biliary cirrhosis (PBC)?

(A) Antimitochondrial antibody (AMA) > 1:40

(B) Hyperlipidemia with elevation of serum unesterified cholesterol

(C) High serum copper levels

(D) Decreased prothrombin time

(E) Sicca syndrome

330. All of the following statements regarding ovarian cancer are true EXCEPT that

(A) it is the most common gynecologic cancer

(B) it has the highest mortality among the common gynecologic cancers

(C) it tends to be asymptomatic until it has reached an advanced stage

(D) its development may be influenced by environmental, cultural, or socioeconomic factors

(E) Pap smears are ineffective for routine diagnostic screening

331. A 70-year-old Irish consular official seeks local medical attention for diarrhea and weight loss, which have been present for 2 years. He says he has always been in good health "even though I'm the runt of the litter" (he is the smallest of eight siblings). Laboratory studies include normal complete blood cell count and serum electrolyte concentrations. Serum D-xylose concentration is 0.76 mmol/L (15 mg/dL) 2 h after an oral challenge, and 24-h fecal fat determination is 12 g with the man on a 100-g fat diet. A representative biopsy specimen of his small bowel is shown below.

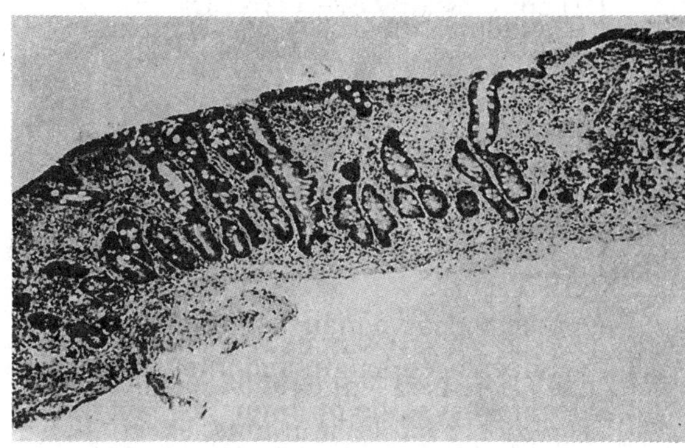

All of the following are true statements about the man's illness EXCEPT

(A) this condition is associated with specific HLA genotypes

(B) abdominal pain, arthralgia, low-grade fever, and lymphadenopathy are frequently present

(C) corticosteroid therapy can reverse jejunal pathology and lessen clinical symptoms

(D) adherence to a strict gluten-free diet usually results in normalization of malabsorption tests and reversal of jejunal pathology

(E) a majority of affected persons complain of bloating after ingesting milk

332. All the following procedures for the detection of cancer for those over age 40 are recommended by the American Cancer Society EXCEPT

(A) yearly mammography (every 1 to 2 years for those 40 to 49 years old)

(B) yearly pelvic examination (with reduction in frequency after three consecutive normal examinations)

(C) yearly Pap smear (with reduction in frequency after three consecutive normal examinations)

(D) yearly digital rectal examination

(E) colonoscopy every 3 years

333. All the following statements regarding physiologic maneuvers used to distinguish one cardiac condition from another are true EXCEPT

(A) the Valsalva maneuver results in a decreased length and intensity for most systolic murmurs, except those due to mitral valve prolapse and hypertrophic cardiomyopathy

(B) in the case of mitral valve prolapse, squatting results in increased intensity of the systolic murmur

(C) handgrip exercise increases the intensity of the murmurs of mitral stenosis and mitral regurgitation

(D) murmurs of tricuspid regurgitation and tricuspid stenosis increase during inspiration

(E) the murmur of aortic stenosis increases following a ventricular premature beat

334. A newborn infant with ambiguous genitalia develops vomiting and profound volume depletion. A diagnosis of congenital adrenal hyperplasia due to C-21 hydroxylase deficiency would NOT be supported by which of the following findings?

(A) Elevated urinary 17-ketosteroid concentration

(B) Elevated plasma 11-deoxycortisol concentration

(C) Elevated plasma 17-hydroxy-progesterone concentration

(D) Elevated plasma androstenedione concentration

(E) Elevated urinary pregnanediol and pregnanetriol concentrations

335. All the following are indications for surgical intervention in the treatment of dissection of the aorta EXCEPT

(A) compromised femoral pulse

(B) involvement of the ascending aorta

(C) involvement of the descending aorta

(D) new murmur of aortic regurgitation

(E) persistent chest pain

336. Which of the following is NOT a major feature (according to the revised Jones criteria) of acute rheumatic fever?

(A) A pink rash with serpiginous margins

(B) Arthritis in both knees

(C) Painless swellings over bony prominences

(D) Pericardial friction rub

(E) Prolonged PR interval

337. All of the following statements are true regarding aortic dissections EXCEPT

(A) type II dissections involve the ascending aorta only

(B) initial medical management includes reduction in myocardial contractility and systemic blood pressure

(C) in-hospital mortality for medically and surgically treated dissections is similar, approximately 15 percent

(D) a bicuspid aortic valve, the most common cardiac anomaly, has been shown to be associated with an increased incidence of aortic dissection

(E) the presence of a pleural effusion suggests a diagnosis other than aortic dissection

338. All of the following techniques are used to evaluate fetal chromosomes EXCEPT

(A) α-fetoprotein level

(B) amniocentesis

(C) cordocentesis

(D) chorionic villous sampling

339. A 50-year-old man with a history of smoking, hypertension, and chronic exertional angina now presents with several daily episodes of chest pain at rest compatible with cardiac ischemia. Which of the following would NOT be included in an appropriate management plan?

(A) Aspirin

(B) Diltiazem

(C) Intravenous heparin

(D) Intravenous nitroglycerin

(E) Lidocaine by bolus infusion

340. Of the following patients, which patient would NOT be at increased risk for the development of deep venous thrombosis?

(A) A 35-year-old woman with systemic lupus erythematosus and a prolonged partial thromboplastin time

(B) A 75-year-old woman with a Colles fracture of the wrist

(C) A normotensive 18-year-old woman taking an oral contraceptive

(D) A 55-year-old man 3 days after an uncomplicated inferior myocardial infarction

(E) A 55-year-old man 5 days after complete resection of a squamous cell carcinoma of 2 cm in diameter in the periphery of the right lung

341. All of the following statements regarding the epidemiology of HIV infection are correct EXCEPT

(A) the occupational risk of HIV infection among health-care workers is small (< 0.5 percent per exposure) but real

(B) over 1 per 1000 U.S. military recruits are infected

(C) most U.S. cases of AIDS are now in the high-risk group of intravenous drug abusers

(D) the chance that a single donor blood unit will contain HIV is between 1:40,000 and 1:250,000

(E) most pediatric cases arise because of in utero transmission from an infected mother

342. Regarding toxoplasmosis in pregnancy, all of the following statements are correct EXCEPT that

(A) it can be acquired by eating infected raw meat

(B) it can be acquired by contact with cat feces

(C) it occurs in 1 in every 2000 to 2500 pregnancies

(D) infection in early pregnancy may lead to abortion

(E) infection in late pregnancy may lead to infection of the fetus

343. All of the following are immunologic abnormalities detected in patients with acquired immunodeficiency syndrome (AIDS) EXCEPT

(A) deficient T-lymphocyte response to antigenic and mitogenic stimulation

(B) decreased serum levels of immunoglobulins

(C) depletion of T4+ lymphocytes

(D) normal numbers of T8+ lymphocytes

(E) defective natural killer cell function

344. A 32-year-old homosexual man complains of weight loss, sweats, diarrhea, and swollen glands for the past 3 to 4 months. Over the previous 1 to 2 months he has had increasing dyspnea and fever and a nonproductive cough. Which of the following pathogens is NOT likely to be associated with this patient's illness?

(A) *Cryptococcus neoformans*

(B) Cytomegalovirus

(C) *Mycobacterium tuberculosis*

(D) *Mycoplasma pneumoniae*

(E) *Pneumocystis carinii*

345. The arthropathy of inflammatory bowel disease is NOT usually characterized by which of the following?

(A) Peripheral arthritis is more commonly associated with colonic than with small-bowel involvement

(B) The presence and activity of the peripheral arthritis is related to the extent and activity of bowel involvement

(C) The peripheral arthritis is usually a symmetrical small-joint polyarthritis

(D) The peripheral arthritis resolves without residual joint damage

(E) Spondylitis is not related to the extent or activity of colonic involvement

346. All of the following groups have an increased risk of infection with *Giardia lamblia* EXCEPT

(A) campers in mountainous areas

(B) male homosexuals

(C) patients receiving chemotherapy

(D) patients with IgA deficiency

(E) toddlers in day-care centers

DIRECTIONS (Questions 347-400): Each set of matching questions in this section consists of a list of four to twenty-six lettered options followed by numbered questions. For each numbered question, select the appropriate lettered option(s). Each lettered option may be used **once, more than once, or not at all.** The question will state the **EXACT NUMBER** of options to select.

Questions 347-348: Match each of the numbered characteristics with the renal tumors listed below.

(A) Angiomyolipoma

(B) Lymphoma

(C) Oncocytoma

(D) Wilms' tumor

347. Bilateral **(SELECT 1 CHOICE)**

348. Spoke-wheel enhancement **(SELECT 1 CHOICE)**

Questions 349-350: Match the side effects below with the appropriate anesthetic.

(A) Enflurane

(B) Halothane

(C) Methoxyflurane

(D) Morphine

(E) Nitrous oxide (N_2O)

349. Nephrotoxicity **(SELECT 1 ANESTHETIC)**

350. Seizures **(SELECT 1 ANESTHETIC)**

Questions 351-352: Match each defect in host immunity with the type of infection most commonly associated with it.

(A) Cytomegalovirus

(B) Gram-negative bacteremia

(C) Recurrent *Neisseria gonorrhoeae* infections

(D) Recurrent staphylococcal skin abscesses

(E) *Streptococcus pneumoniae* bacteremia

351. Deficiencies of late complement components **(SELECT 1 INFECTION)**

352. Postsplenectomy state **(SELECT 1 INFECTION)**

Questions 353-354: Match the gastrointestinal content at each site with its appropriate ionic composition (meq/L).

	Na^+	K^+	Cl^-	HCO_3^-
(A)	140	5	104	30
(B)	140	5	75	115
(C)	60	10	130	0
(D)	10	26	10	30
(E)	60	30	40	50

353. Salivary **(SELECT 1 CHOICE)**

354. Stomach **(SELECT 1 CHOICE)**

Questions 355-357: A teenager with new onset seizures is to start anti-convulsant therapy. She has concerns about the potential side effects. For each systemic side effect listed below, choose the anticonvulsant drug with which it is most likely to be associated.

(A) Carbamazepine

(B) Clonazepam

(C) Phenobarbital

(D) Phenytoin

(E) Valproic acid

355. Hirsutism **(SELECT 1 DRUG)**

356. Gum hyperplasia **(SELECT 1 DRUG)**

357. Leukopenia **(SELECT 1 DRUG)**

Questions 358-359: Select the appropriate interspace level for the following neurologic findings associated with sciatica.

(A) L2-L3 interspace

(B) L3-L4 interspace

(C) L4-L5 interspace

(D) L5-S1 interspace

(E) S1-S2 interspace

358. Inability to walk on toes and depressed ankle tendon reflex **(SELECT 1 LEVEL)**

359. Foot-drop with normal reflexes **(SELECT 1 LEVEL)**

Questions 360-361: For each of the numbered patients below, select the ultrasonic finding of most concern.

(A) Fetal ascites

(B) Malposition of the placenta

(C) Short femur length

(D) Spinal defects

(E) Twins

360. A patient is 20 weeks pregnant by her last menstrual period but measures 30 cm in fundal height **(SELECT 1 FINDING)**

361. A patient is 24 weeks pregnant and is seen after an episode of heavy bleeding per vagina **(SELECT 1 FINDING)**

Questions 362-363: Match each of the numbered chemotherapeutic agents to its appropriate mechanism of action.

(A) Binds with DNA and causes untwisting of the double helix

(B) Blocks thymidylate synthetase

(C) Causes depurination and miscoding errors by its alkylating action

(D) Inhibits DNA synthesis and reacts with DNA to cause strand scission

(E) Produces metaphase arrest by direct binding to tubulin

362. Bleomycin **(SELECT 1 MECHANISM)**

363. Doxorubicin **(SELECT 1 MECHANISM)**

Questions 364-365: Match each numbered drug or characteristic with the appropriate form of esophagitis.

(A) *Candida*

(B) *Herpes simplex* virus

(C) Pill-induced

(D) Radiation

364. Tetracycline **(SELECT 1 FORM)**

365. Punched-out superficial ulcers **(SELECT 1 FORM)**

Questions 366-368: Match each numbered description with the correct type of abortion.

(A) Complete abortion

(B) Incomplete abortion

(C) Inevitable abortion

(D) Missed abortion

(E) Threatened abortion

366. Uterine bleeding at 12 weeks' gestation accompanied by cervical dilation without passage of tissue **(SELECT 1 TYPE)**

367. Passage of some but not all placental tissue through the cervix at 9 weeks' gestation **(SELECT 1 TYPE)**

368. Fetal death at 15 weeks' gestation without expulsion of any fetal or maternal tissue for at least 8 weeks **(SELECT 1 TYPE)**

Questions 369-370: Match each of the following numbered polyposis syndromes to its corresponding feature.

(A) Adenoma

(B) Brain tumor

(C) Hamartoma

(D) Osteoma

369. Familial colonic polyposis **(SELECT 1 FEATURE)**

370. Gardner's **(SELECT 1 FEATURE)**

Questions 371-372: Match each of the numbered causes of right heart failure below with the most characteristic set of hemodynamic measurements.

	Right atrial pressure, mmHg	**Pulmonary arterial pressure, mmHg**	**Pulmonary capillary wedge pressure, mmHg**
(A)	16	75/30	11
(B)	16	35/17	16
(C)	16	100/30	28
(D)	16	45/22	20
(E)	16	22/12	10
Normal values	0-5	12-28/3-13	3-11

371. Right ventricular infarction **(SELECT 1 SET)**

372. Cor pulmonale from bronchitis **(SELECT 1 SET)**

Questions 373-374: Match the numbered hepatobiliary abnormality with the most appropriate nuclear medicine study listed below.

(A) Iminoacetic acid cholecystectomy

(B) Labeled red blood cells (RBC)

(C) Sulfur colloid

(D) Xenon

373. Bile peritonitis following laparoscopy **(SELECT 1 STUDY)**

374. Cavernous hemangioma **(SELECT 1 STUDY)**

Questions 375-376: There are several mechanisms that affect blood clotting. Match the following tests with the coagulation mechanism they most specifically evaluate.

(A) Extrinsic pathway

(B) Fibrinogen function

(C) Intrinsic pathway

(D) Platelet function

(E) None of the above

375. Bleeding time **(SELECT 1 CHOICE)**

376. Thrombin time **(SELECT 1 CHOICE)**

Questions 377-378: Match the following pancreatic endocrine tumors with the clinical features listed below.

(A) Beta cell tumor

(B) Cholera-like symptoms

(C) Delta cell tumor

(D) Hyperglycemia

(E) Wheezing

377. Carcinoid **(SELECT 1 FEATURE)**

378. Gastrinoma **(SELECT 1 FEATURE)**

Questions 379-380: For each of the numbered syndromes or diseases below, choose the virus responsible when the fetus is exposed in utero.

(A) Cytomegalovirus

(B) Hepatitis B

(C) Rubella

(D) Rubeola

(E) Varicella zoster

379. Cataracts, cardiac defects, deafness **(SELECT 1 VIRUS)**

380. Cirrhosis, primary hepatocellular carcinoma **(SELECT 1 VIRUS)**

Questions 381-382: Match the following numbered hereditary syndromes with the associated tumors.

(A) Glioblastoma

(B) Leukemia

(C) Renal cell carcinoma

(D) Rhabdomyoma

381. Ataxia-telangiectasia **(SELECT 1 TUMOR)**

382. Neurofibromatosis **(SELECT 1 TUMOR)**

Questions 383-384: For each of the disorders below, select the characteristic hemodynamic pattern.

(A) Dip-and-plateau pattern

(B) Equalization of diastolic pressures

(C) Slow *y* descent

(D) Tall *v* wave

(E) None of the above

383. Pericardial tamponade
(SELECT 1 CHOICE)

384. Amyloidosis
(SELECT 1 CHOICE)

Questions 385-386: For each description below, select the type of fracture or dislocation with which is it most likely to be associated.

(A) Greenstick fracture

(B) Monteggia's deformity

(C) Navicular fracture

(D) Posterior shoulder dislocation

(E) Spiral fracture

385. Associated with seizure
(SELECT 1 CHOICE)

386. May result in avascular neurosis
(SELECT 1 CHOICE)

Questions 387-388: For each syndrome below, select the associated cardiovascular abnormality.

(A) Coarctation of the aorta

(B) Cor pulmonale

(C) Endocardial cushion defect

(D) Mitral regurgitation

(E) Pulmonic stenosis

387. Marfan's syndrome
(SELECT 1 ABNORMALITY)

388. Turner's syndrome
(SELECT 1 ABNORMALITY)

Questions 389-390: Match the descriptions below with the appropriate infectious agent or condition.

(A) Atrophic (senile) vaginitis

(B) *Candida albicans*

(C) *Gardnerella vaginalis* (formerly *Haemophilus vaginalis*)

(D) *Neisseria gonorrhoeae*

(E) *Trichomonas vaginalis*

389. A frequent cause of nonspecific vaginitis
(SELECT 1 CHOICE)

390. Diabetes mellitus may be a predisposing factor **(SELECT 1 CHOICE)**

Questions 391-392: Match the following numbered red blood cell morphologies with the associated disorder.

(A) Autoimmune hemolytic anemia

(B) Prosthetic heart valve

(C) Severe liver disease

(D) Thallasemia

391. Acanthocytes **(SELECT 1 CHOICE)**

392. Schistocytes **(SELECT 1 CHOICE)**

Questions 393-394: Match the following disease entities with the ultrasound appearance most closely associated.

(A) Large, echogenic kidneys

(B) Noncommunicating cystic structures in a single kidney

(C) Communicating cystic structures

(D) Small echogenic kidneys

(E) Large hypoechoic kidneys

393. Infantile polycystic kidney disease **(SELECT 1 CHOICE)**

394. Multicystic dysplastic kidney **(SELECT 1 CHOICE)**

Questions 395-396: Match each of the numbered malignancies with the appropriate cells or cellular characteristics.

(A) Cytoplasmic extensions

(B) Langerhan's cells

(C) Osteoclast-activating factor

(D) Reed-Sternberg cell

395. Myeloma **(SELECT 1 CHOICE)**

396. Hairy cell leukemia **(SELECT 1 CHOICE)**

Questions 397-398: For each of the following patterns of chest x-ray and clinical presentation, select the cardiac condition with which it is most closely associated.

(A) Increased pulmonary blood flow with cyanosis

(B) Decreased pulmonary blood flow with cyanosis

(C) Increased pulmonary blood flow without cyanosis

(D) Decreased pulmonary blood flow without cyanosis

(E) Normal pulmonary blood flow with cyanosis

397. Complete transposition of the great vessels **(SELECT 1 CONDITION)**

398. Sinus venosus atrial septal defect **(SELECT 1 CONDITION)**

Questions 399-400: Match the numbered chemotherapeutic agents with their most common side effects.

(A) Cardiac toxicity

(B) Hemorrhagic cystitis

(C) Necrotizing enterocolitis

(D) Ocular degeneration

(E) Pancreatic failure

(F) Peripheral neuropathy

(G) Pulmonary fibrosis

(H) Renal failure

(I) Tympanic membrane fibrosis

399. Cyclophosphamide
(SELECT 1 SIDE EFFECT)

400. Cisplatin
(SELECT 1 SIDE EFFECT)

STOP. You have completed this PreTest Examination. Go back over your answers and be sure your answer sheet is carefully marked.

Book A

Correct Answers

Number of items: 200

1. CLINICAL THERAPEUTICS: CONTINUED CARE: ANSWER: B
(Isselbacher, 13/e, chaps 45, 236.) In a cirrhotic patient, massive extracellular volume expansion and low urine sodium excretion are evidence of inappropriate sodium retention. If serum creatinine concentration is elevated in addition, the possibility of incipient renal failure—the so-called hepatorenal syndrome—should be entertained. Attempts at rapid volume reduction in this setting can precipitate renal failure and thus are contraindicated. Current treatment recommendations call for rest, observation, a possible trial of plasma expansion, and then gentle diuresis if renal function remains stable.

2. APPLYING BASIC CONCEPTS: CONTINUED CARE: ANSWER: E
(Carr, pp 49-51, 60-63.) The appearance of breast buds, thelarche, is the first sign of puberty and is usually seen between the ages of 9 and 11. This is subsequently followed by pubarche, the adolescent growth spurt, and finally menarche. If thelarche has not occurred by the age of 13, or menarche by the age of 15, the patient should be fully evaluated for delayed sexual development.

3. DIAGNOSIS: EMERGENCY: ANSWER: E
(Wilmore, vol 1, sect 1, chap 5, pp 5-7.) The patient presented in the question is in a state of metabolic acidosis as shown by a markedly increased anion gap of 28 meq unmeasured anions per liter of plasma. However, the respiratory response is greater than can be explained by a compensatory response, since the patient is mildly alkalemic. The disturbance cannot be a pure respiratory alkalosis, since the serum bicarbonate does not drop below 15 meq/L as a result of renal compensation, and the anion gap does not vary more than 1 to 2 meq/L from its normal value of 12 in response to a respiratory disturbance. The renal response to hyperventilation involves wasting of bicarbonate and compensatory retention of chloride; it does not involve a change in the concentration of "unmeasured" anions.

4. DIAGNOSIS: EMERGENCY: ANSWER: A
(Anderson, Ann Intern Med 85:745-748, 1976. Isselbacher, 13/e, pp 2458-2459.) The acid-base disturbance in the patient described in the previous question demonstrates the value of extracting all available information from a small amount of rapidly retrievable data—e.g, arterial blood gases. Salicylates directly stimulate the respiratory center and produce respiratory alkalosis. By building up an accumulation of organic acids, salicylates also produce a concomitant metabolic acidosis. Characteristically both disturbances exist simultaneously following massive ingestion of salicylates. If sedative agents have been taken as well, the respiratory alkalosis (and even the respiratory compensation) may be absent. Phenformin and methanol overdoses also produce "high anion-gap" metabolic acidosis, but without the simultaneous respiratory disturbance. In the case presented, the patient's history of tinnitus in conjunction with his mixed metabolic acidosis-respiratory alkalosis is essentially pathognomonic of salicylate intoxication.

5. CLINICAL THERAPEUTICS: CONTINUED CARE: ANSWER: C
(Schwartz, 6/e, pp 65-66.) A ruptured abdominal aneurysm is a surgical emergency often accompanied by serious hypotension and vascular collapse before surgery and massive fluid shifts with renal failure after surgery. In this case, all the hemodynamic parameters indicate inadequate intravascular volume, and the patient is therefore suffering from hypovolemic hypotension. The low urine output indicates poor renal perfusion, while the high urine specific gravity indicates adequate renal function with compensatory free water conservation. The administration of a vasopressor agent would certainly raise the blood

pressure, but it would do so by increasing peripheral vascular resistance and thereby further decrease tissue perfusion. The deleterious effects of shock would be increased. A vasodilating agent to lower the systemic vascular resistance would lead to profound hypotension and possibly complete vascular collapse because of pooling of an already depleted vascular volume. This patient's blood pressure is critically dependent on an elevated systemic vascular resistance. To properly treat this patient, rapid fluid infusion and expansion of the intravascular volume must be undertaken. This can be easily done with lactated Ringer's solution or blood (or both) until improvements in such parameters as the pulmonary capillary wedge pressure, urine output, and blood pressure are noted.

6. DIAGNOSTIC STUDIES: CONTINUED CARE: ANSWER: C
(Isselbacher, 13/e, chap 247.) The most important differential diagnosis in the case presented is between a renal cell carcinoma and a benign cystic lesion. Urinalysis may be normal in the presence of renal cell carcinoma, and urinary cytology is unfortunately of little value in the diagnosis of this lesion. Ultrasonography will reveal whether or not the lesion is cystic. If the lesion appears cystic on both IVP and ultrasonographic examination and the patient does not have hematuria, the cyst can be considered benign with a diagnostic accuracy of 97 percent. If greater assurance is required or if there are changes on follow-up radiologic studies, then needle aspiration should be carried out. If the ultrasound appearance is not consistent with a simple cyst, then contrast-enhanced CT scanning, the optimal test for diagnosis and staging of renal cell carcinoma, should be performed.

7. CLINICAL INTERVENTION: CONTINUED CARE: ANSWER: E
(Isselbacher, 13/e, pp 1336-1338.) The accuracy of ultrasound in the diagnosis of a 3-cm renal cyst is nearly 100 percent. No further imaging or treatment is necessary. Renal cysts are very common in the adult population and should not be implicated as the source of hypertension or connote an underlying cystic disease.

8. PROGNOSIS: INITIAL WORKUP: ANSWER: D
(Isselbacher, 13/e, pp 1295-1297.) The proteinuria of acute glomerular nephritis is usually moderate but can be as high as 3 gm/day and result in nephrotic syndrome. Direct damage to the glomerular wall or peritubular capillaries allows erythrocytes to cross into the filtrate and results in a gross hematuria often described as cola- or coffee-colored urine. Leukocytes can also cross into the filtrate and leukocyte casts are common in acute glomerular nephritis. The course of acute glomerular nephritis is usually self-limited, especially in children who contract the disease in the epidemic form, but can progress to an acute sustained renal failure in a matter of weeks. Renal biopsy in this group of patients will often show a cresentic glomerulonephritis.

9. PROGNOSIS: EMERGENCY: ANSWER: E
(Davis, pp 2350-2351.) Median nerve injury at the wrist level results in paralysis of the thenar muscles that position the thumb for opposition to the other fingers. A clawhand and paralysis of intrinsic flexor hand muscles indicate a problem associated with ulnar nerve injury; a wristdrop results from radial nerve injury.

10. HEALTH MAINTENANCE: CONTINUED CARE: ANSWER: B

(Jones, 4/e, pp 298-303.) Achondroplasia is associated with an autosomal dominant pattern of inheritance. However, mutation accounts for 90 percent of all cases of the disorder. Affected women almost always require cesarean section because of the distorted shape of their pelves. Women who have achondroplasia and receive adequate treatment for its associated complications, including the neurologic signs of cord compression due to spinal deformity, generally have a normal life expectancy.

11. DIAGNOSIS: INITIAL WORKUP: ANSWER: A

(Isselbacher, 13/e, chap 45.) The differential diagnosis of hyponatremia depends on exclusion of artifactual causes followed by an assessment of volume status. Artifactual hyponatremia can occur in the setting of hyperlipidemia (where a portion of any volume of plasma taken for analysis will be sodium-free lipid) or extreme hyperproteinemia (plasma proteins occupy more than the normal 7 percent of plasma volume) as in multiple myeloma. In these cases plasma osmolality should not be depressed. Actually, modern sodium-selective electrodes eliminate artifactual hyponatremia by measuring the sodium concentration in plasma volume only, not total plasma volume.

In diabetes with very high blood sugars, plasma osmolality may actually be increased in the face of significant hyponatremia. Plasma sodium can become diluted by the movement of water outside cells in the presence of any osmotically active solute. For every elevation of 5.5 mmol/L (100 mg/dL) of plasma glucose, plasma sodium will decrease by 1.6 mmol/L.

In congestive heart failure or any edema-forming state in which the "effective" arterial blood volume is depressed, hyponatremia may ensue. This situation is generally accompanied by alkalosis and hypokalemia because mineralocorticoid secretion is high. On the other hand, acidosis and hyperkalemia would be associated with the hyponatremia of Addison's disease (adrenal insufficiency) with insufficient aldosterone present to cause the distal tubular reabsorption of sodium bicarbonate and the concomitant extrusion of potassium chloride.

The inappropriate secretion of vasopressin, or ADH (SIADH), may occur in multiple settings including head trauma, drug use (vincristine, narcotics), pain, or bacterial meningitis. Vasopressin has little effect on the renal excretion of potassium and hydrogen ions. Patients with SIADH must be euvolemic. Thus, hyponatremia in this setting is usually not accompanied by changes in concentrations of BUN or creatinine (if anything, they are low-normal), potassium, or bicarbonate.

12. PROGNOSIS: INITIAL WORKUP: ANSWER: C

(Isselbacher, 13/e, pp 1337-1338.) 50 percent of patients with renal cell carcinoma will have anemia at presentation; only 10 percent will have erythrocytosis due to erythropoietin production by the tumor. Invasion of the left renal vein with tumor thrombus can cause obstruction of the left gonadal vein (which drains into the left renal vein) and subsequent varicocele. This will raise the stage of the tumor to III but does not preclude resection. Tumor thrombus can be excised if it is in continuity with the primary tumor—even if it extends into the IVC or right atrium. Von Hippel-Lindau disease is associated with a high incidence of renal tumors including renal cell carcinoma which is frequently bilateral. Screening studies, ultrasound or CT, are useful in early detection of these solid tumors when partial nephrectomy can be achieved to preserve as much renal tissue as possible. The majority of renal cell carcinomas contain dystrophic calcifications, frequently visible on plain films and CT. The presence of distant metastases, stage IV, reduces the 5-year survival rate from 15 to 50 percent to less than 5 percent.

13. CLINICAL INTERVENTION: EMERGENCY: ANSWER: C

(Isselbacher, 13/e, chap 217.) Several investigators have shown that the most efficient means of assessing the severity of an asthmatic attack and of following the therapeutic response is the measure-

ment of some parameter of respiratory function such as peak flow or forced expiratory volume in 1 s (FEV_1). The chest radiograph will frequently show only hyperinflation in attacks of varying degrees of severity. Arterial blood gases will reflect hypoxemia and hypocapnia in all but the most severe episodes, when they may reflect respiratory fatigue and severe obstruction as rising P_{CO_2} levels. Accessory muscle use and the presence of pulsus paradoxus reflect changes in intrathoracic pressure and the work of breathing, and they may actually disappear if the patient's breathing worsens to the point of becoming shallow. Thus, these signs may be misleading.

14. DIAGNOSTIC STUDIES: EMERGENCY: ANSWER: A
(Schwartz, 6/e, pp 199-201.) The "coiled spring" appearance of the duodenum in the setting of trauma is due to an intramural hematoma which can cause partial or complete obstruction of the intestine. It presents as a high bowel obstruction with abdominal pain and occasionally a palpable right upper quadrant mass. An upper gastrointestinal series is almost always diagnostic with the classic coiled spring appearance of the second and third portions of the duodenum secondary to the crowding of the valvulae conniventes (circular folds) by the hematoma.

15. CLINICAL INTERVENTION: EMERGENCY: ANSWER: D
(Schwartz, 6/e, pp 199-201.) Nonsurgical management is the mainstay of therapy as the vast majority of duodenal hematomas resolve spontaneously. Simple evacuation of the hematoma is the operative procedure of choice. However, bypass procedures and duodenal resection have been performed for this problem. In patients with duodenal obstruction from the superior mesenteric artery syndrome, the obstruction is usually the result of a marked weight loss and, in conjunction with this, loss of the retroperitoneal fat pad that elevates the superior mesenteric artery from the third and fourth portions of the duodenum. Nutritional repletion and replenishment of this fat pad will elevate the artery off the duodenum and relieve the obstruction.

16. CLINICAL INTERVENTION: CONTINUED CARE: ANSWER: E
(Eden, pp 269-276. Evans, pp 225-229.) The recommended sequence for an MSAFP screening program for a thousand hypothetical patients would normally produce about 40 with an elevated level (2.5 multiples of the median—MOM) on the first MSAFP. If the patient does not have an extremely elevated value (i.e., the value is <4.0 MOM) and is relatively early (<19 weeks' gestation), a second MSAFP value is usually drawn. About two-thirds of these patients will have an elevated test or will be very high the first time. Those that are normal a second time drop back into the normal population. However, if the value is extremely high (≥4.0 MOM) or if the gestational age is approaching the limit of options for termination of pregnancy (19+ weeks), most programs then skip a second test and go directly on to ultrasound and possibly amniocentesis. A thorough ultrasound on patients with two elevations or one very high elevation will reveal an obvious reason for the elevation in about 10 of 30 patients. These reasons may include anencephaly, twins, wrong gestational age of the fetus, or a fetal demise. About 20 patients with no obvious cause for their elevation should then be offered counseling and amniocentesis. Of these 20, about 1 or 2 will have an elevated amniotic fluid alpha-fetoprotein and positive acetylcholinesterase. Such patients will have a greater than 99 percent chance of having a baby with an open neural tube defect or other serious malformations, such as a ventral wall defect. Amniography is an outmoded procedure in which radiopaque dye is injected into the amniotic cavity for the purpose of taking x-rays. Under no circumstances whatsoever should termination of pregnancy be recommended on the basis of MSAFP testing alone. MSAFP is only a screening test used to define who is at risk and requires further testing; it is never diagnostic.

17. DIAGNOSIS: CONTINUED CARE: ANSWER: E
(Isselbacher, 13/e, chap 238.) In the first week after renal transplantation, the differential diagnosis of graft dysfunction includes early rejection, hypovolemia, cyclosporine intoxication, acute tubular necrosis, urinary obstruction, and renal artery thrombosis. Cyclosporine can mask many of the classic signs of rejection, such as fever and graft tenderness; renal biopsy is often needed to make the diagnosis. However, renal ultrasonography should precede any manipulation to rule out mechanical outflow obstruction, as it should in any patient with acute deterioration of renal function.

18. DIAGNOSTIC STUDIES: CONTINUED CARE: ANSWER: C
(Isselbacher, 13/e, chap 225. Rich, Prog Cardiovasc Dis 31:205, 1988.) Primary pulmonary hypertension is an uncommon disease that usually affects young women. Early in the illness affected persons often are diagnosed as psychoneurotic because of the vague nature of presenting complaints—for example, dyspnea, chest pain, and evidence of hyperventilation without hypoxemia on arterial blood-gas testing. However, progression of the disease leads to syncope in approximately one-half of cases and signs of right heart failure on physical examination. Chest x-ray typically shows enlarged central pulmonary arteries with or without attenuation of peripheral markings. The diagnosis of primary pulmonary hypertension is made by documentation of elevated pressures by right heart catheterization and by exclusion of other pathologic processes. Lung disease of sufficient severity to cause pulmonary hypertension would be evident by history and on examination. Major differential diagnoses include thromboemboli and heart disease; outside the United States, schistosomiasis and filariasis are common causes of pulmonary hypertension, and a careful travel history should be taken.

19. CLINICAL THERAPEUTICS: CONTINUED CARE: ANSWER: A
(Isselbacher, 13/e, chap 218.) Given the temporal relationship of the symptoms to the work with rats, serologic evidence for inflammation, the nonspecific radiographic findings, and the restrictive pulmonary physiology suggested by spirographic examination, the most likely diagnosis is acute hypersensitivity pneumonitis with male rat urine probably the offending antigen. Without treatment, the patient could develop the subacute or chronic form of the disease with potentially serious physiologic impairment. While steroids can be helpful in severe or chronic cases, the best therapy is to remove the offending antigen or to remove the patient from an environment where exposure is inevitable. This approach is difficult when the patient's lifestyle or livelihood requires a radical change; in the case presented, however, simply restricting the student's laboratory efforts to those not involving direct animal care seems relatively nondisruptive.

20. DIAGNOSTIC STUDIES: CONTINUED CARE: ANSWER: A
(Isselbacher, 13/e, chap 218. Greenberger, Chest 91:1655, 1987.) Allergic bronchopulmonary aspergillosis is a hypersensitivity pneumonitis involving an allergic reaction to antigens from the Aspergillus species, most commonly *A. fumigatus*. The diagnosis should be suspected in asthmatic persons who have recurrent pulmonary infiltrates associated with peripheral blood or sputum eosinophilia. Suggestive laboratory findings include serum immunoglobulin E levels elevated many times above normal and the presence of aspergilli in the sputum. Antigenic skin testing is positive both in immediate (type I, wheal and flare) reaction and reaction evident after 4 to 6 h (type III, erythema and induration). Delayed, tuberculin-type (type IV, cell-mediated) reactions, however, do not occur. Serum precipitins to aspergilli are found in a majority of affected persons. The inflammatory response leads to dilatation of central airways and often is evident radiographically as mucoid impaction.

21. DIAGNOSIS: EMERGENCY: ANSWER: B
(Isselbacher, 13/e, chaps 218, 224.) Chronic eosinophilic pneumonia is an interstitial lung disorder of unknown cause that produces a systemic illness characterized by fever, weight loss, and malaise. Although lung biopsy shows an eosinophilic infiltrate involving both the interstitium and the alveolar space, there may not be an associated eosinophilia in the peripheral blood. The diagnosis should be suggested by the "photonegative pulmonary edema" pattern, with central sparing and nonsegmental, patchy infiltrates in the lung periphery. This disorder often responds dramatically to corticosteroid therapy. Idiopathic pulmonary fibrosis and polymyositis produce diffuse reticular, nodular, or reticulonodular infiltrates on chest x-ray. Alveolar proteinosis is a rare disorder that most often produces a diffuse air-space filling pattern radiating from hilar regions on chest x-ray, often with air bronchograms. Alveolar proteinosis does not cause fever unless complicated by infection such as nocardiosis. Lymphangiomyomatosis is also rare. It occurs exclusively in women of childbearing age. The chest x-ray shows reticulonodular infiltration but the lungs often appear hyperinflated. Lymphangiomyomatosis is complicated by pleural effusion and pneumothorax, but not fever.

22. HEALTH MAINTENANCE: CONTINUED CARE: ANSWER: C
(Carr, pp 592-593, 602-605.) At the present time, radiologic screening techniques for osteoporosis in all patients are controversial. X-rays will pick up fractures and bone abnormalities but will miss osteoporosis unless a significant amount of bone loss is already present. Single-photon absorptiometry is accurate in predicting bone loss in the radius; however, it has decreased sensitivity in relation to the axial skeleton. Dual-photon absorptiometry is more accurate in this regard. At the present time it is thought that, for women who are reluctant to use estrogen in the menopausal period, dual-photon absorptiometry or quantitative computed tomography may be used to document rapid bone loss and determine whether the patient is at significant risk of developing fractures. These tests are not screening tools to be used on all menopausal patients.

23. APPLYING BASIC CONCEPTS: CONTINUED CARE: ANSWER: D
(Isselbacher, 13/e, chap 230.) With mild respiratory distress syndrome, or early in the clinical picture, ventilation-perfusion abnormalities are primarily responsible for hypoxemia; therefore, modest increases in the inspired oxygen tension would produce significant increases in arterial oxygenation. As the disease becomes fully developed, however, diffuse alveolar collapse occurs, and right-to-left shunts are created. Under these circumstances, hypoxemia would be insensitive to small changes in inspired oxygen concentration.

24. CLINICAL INTERVENTION: CONTINUED CARE: ANSWER: E
(Isselbacher, 13/e, chaps 230, 231.) Some persons who become agitated or anxious while on a mechanical ventilator receive inadequate ventilation because they are breathing out of phase with the machine. The woman described in the question has adequate oxygenation—a P_{O_2} of 70 mmHg means her hemoglobin is more than 90 percent saturated. However, she is hypoventilating and has developed an acute respiratory acidosis. Positive end-expiratory pressure (PEEP) improves oxygenation by raising the lung volume and reducing shunting but it does not have a large effect on carbon dioxide clearance. Therefore, the appropriate first step in management would be to administer a sedative and control the woman's ventilation, in order to reduce arterial P_{CO_2} and raise pH.

25. HEALTH MAINTENANCE: CONTINUED CARE: ANSWER: C

(Schwartz, 5/e, p 332.) There has been a steady increase in the death rate from lung cancer in this country since 1930. The rate has gone from 18 to 67 per 100,000 in men and from 4.6 to 16.6 per 100,000 in women. Over that time span, there has been a drastic decrease in the death rate from stomach and uterine cancer; this decrease has been attributed to improved surveillance and therapy. There has been a mild increase in both the incidence and mortality of pancreatic cancer. Breast cancer and colon cancer death rates have been stable over the last 40 years.

26. APPLYING BASIC CONCEPTS: CONTINUED CARE: ANSWER: E

(Isselbacher, 13/e, chap 375. Gabuzda, Ann Intern Med 107:383, 1987.) Infected macrophages are probably the Trojan horse by which the human immunodeficiency virus (HIV) enters the central nervous system. AIDS dementia, which is the chief manifestation of subacute encephalitis, the most common neurologic abnormality in this group of patients, is insidious and slowly progressive. The initial CT or MRI scan is normal; the CSF is nonspecifically abnormal (mild pleocytosis and protein rise). Zidovudine (AZT) may be effective if given early in this tragic complication of HIV infection. CNS toxoplasmosis or lymphoma, occurring as a result of the immunocompromised state, can produce mass lesions in AIDS patients. Direct HIV infection is also responsible for the myelopathy, neuropathy, and aseptic meningitis that occur in AIDS patients.

27. DIAGNOSTIC STUDIES: CONTINUED CARE: ANSWER: B

(Schwartz, 6/e, pp 1629-1633.) The thyroid scan illustrated in the question shows a single focus of increased isotope uptake, often referred to as a "hot" nodule; the remainder of the thyroid gland has not taken up radioactive iodine. Hyperfunctioning adenomas become independent of thyroid stimulating hormone (TSH) control and secrete thyroid hormone autonomously, which results in clinical hyperthyroidism. The elevated thyroid hormone levels ultimately diminish TSH levels severely and thus depress function of the remaining normal thyroid gland. An isolated focus of increased uptake on a thyroid scan is virtually diagnostic of a hyperfunctioning adenoma. Carcinomas usually display diminished uptake and are called "cold" nodules. Graves' disease would probably manifest as a diffusely hyperactive gland without nodularity. Multinodular goiter would display many nodules with varying activity.

28. HISTORY AND PHYSICAL: CONTINUED CARE: ANSWER: A

(Isselbacher, 13/e, chap 372. Tandan, Ann Neurol 18:271, 1985.) Amyotrophic lateral sclerosis (ALS) is an untreatable disease that results in progressive loss of upper and lower motor neuron function. Other components of the nervous system remain intact, including the neurons required for ocular motility. Limb weakness and cramping is the first symptom, followed by muscular atrophy, fasciculations, and loss of function of cranial nerve musculature. Early in the disease, upper-tract signs may predominate, resulting in spasticity. Pneumonia due to failure of clearance of secretions is usually the terminal event. Treatable causes of motor neuron disease, such as cervical spondylosis (no bulbar involvement) and lead poisoning, should be excluded whenever the diagnosis of ALS is considered. Guillain-Barré syndrome produces an ascending, rapidly developing paralysis. B_{12} deficiency should lead to abnormalities in posterior column function. Lambert-Eaton syndrome is a paraneoplastic neuromuscular disorder that would not feature upper-tract signs.

29. HEALTH MAINTENANCE: CONTINUED CARE: ANSWER: A
(Schwartz, Surg Gynecol Obstet 166:6-10, 1988.) In a review of 1132 patients who underwent biopsy of occult breast lesions, irrespective of the specific mammographic indication for biopsy (clustered microcalcification, mass, or density distortion), no patient (n = 126) with noninvasive or microinvasive carcinoma had axillary metastasis. When invasive carcinoma was found on the breast biopsy, 33 percent had lymph nodes with metastases.

30. PROGNOSIS: CONTINUED CARE: ANSWER: D
(Barron, pp 42-47.) The glomerular filtration rate (GFR) increases early in pregnancy—by as much as 50 percent by the beginning of the second trimester. The elevated GFR persists to term. The precise mechanism has not been identified.

31. HISTORY AND PHYSICAL: EMERGENCY: ANSWER: B
(Isselbacher, 13/e, chap 14.) The patient had cluster headache. Cluster headache occurs over the orbit, usually within 2 h of falling asleep. The key to diagnosis is a history of associated lacrimation, nasal stuffiness, and swelling and erythema over the cheek. The headaches may occur every night for weeks and are quite severe. Ergotamine taken at bedtime is often the first preparation to prevent the headache. Lithium is frequently effective, but its use warrants monitoring of the patient's serum electrolytes and renal function. Alcohol frequently precipitates headache in these patients. Note that the dose of ergotamine in Choice D is dangerously excessive. Ergotamine should be limited to a maximum of about 12 mg per week.

32. DIAGNOSIS: INITIAL WORKUP: ANSWER: D
(Isselbacher, 13/e, chap 370. Martin, N Engl J Med 315:1267, 1986.) Huntington's chorea, which is inherited as an autosomal dominant trait, is characterized by dementia and choreiform movements. The motor disorder may include grimacing, respiratory spasms, speech irregularity, and a dancing, jangling quality of the gait. Laboratory workup is normal except that atrophy of the caudate may be seen on a carefully evaluated CT or MRI scan. Through the use of DNA linkage analysis, patients can be tested before disease development, if this is appropriate from a psychosocial standpoint.

33. CLINICAL INTERVENTION: CONTINUED CARE: ANSWER: B
(Isselbacher, 13/e, chap 15.) Malignancy in the pelvis frequently causes compression or infiltration of nerves exiting the spinal cord en route to the leg. This results in stepwise progression of sensory and motor deficits in areas supplied by the involved nerve roots or trunks. Continuous pain in the distribution of a specific nerve or root is also common. In this patient the neurologic deficits began in an Sl distribution but then progressed to L5 and, finally, L4 roots, suggesting an expanding paravertebral mass. Isolated, spontaneous activity of muscle fibers called fibrillations is characteristic of denervation. Nerve conduction will be normal in the leg if the lesion is proximal to the measuring electrodes, i.e., in the pelvis. An expanding cortical mass might also cause progressive numbness in the foot and leg and might be missed on a CT scan that does not take cuts all the way up to the vertex. Back pain and neuropathic pain would not occur with a cortical lesion, and the reflexes under such circumstances should be hyperactive.

34. DIAGNOSIS: INITIAL WORKUP: ANSWER: D

(Schwartz, 5/e, pp 563-564.) A subareolar tender lump associated with a bloody nipple discharge is a classic presentation for intraductal papilloma. Papillomas are benign proliferations of the epithelium that line the large lactiferous ducts beneath the nipple. The lesions usually are palpable as discrete, small, often tender masses, which usually are freely movable, although secondary infection and fibrosis may cause fixation to adjacent tissue. Since cancer occasionally presents with signs and symptoms indistinguishable from those of a ductal papilloma, excisional biopsy should always be done. If an intraductal papilloma is found, excision suffices for therapy.

35. DIAGNOSIS: CONTINUED CARE: ANSWER: E

(Isselbacher, 13/e, chap 376.) The cause of chronic subdural hematoma may be a trivial or unapparent injury, such as might be sustained by a sudden deceleration experienced in a motor vehicle accident. Symptoms are relatively nonspecific, usually characterized by an intermittent headache accompanied by some degree of personality change, drowsiness, or confusion. This condition is easily confused with drug intoxication, stroke, dementia, and depression. For the patient in the question, however, the lack of focal findings argues against stroke and the rapidity of onset would be unusual for dementia. The CT scan does not define the hematomas because they have become isodense with the passage of time (2 to 6 weeks since injury); however, the absence of sulci and the small size of the ventricles coupled with the clinical scenario are highly suggestive of bilateral subdural hematomas. Surgical evacuation of the hematomas is the treatment of choice.

36. PROGNOSIS: CONTINUED CARE: ANSWER: D

(Burrow, 3/e, pp 148-150.) The overall incidence of neural tube defects in the United States is 1 to 2 per 1000 live births. However, a mother with a previous child with a neural tube defect has a recurrent risk ranging from 1.7 to 6 percent. Levels of alpha-fetoprotein in maternal serum vary with gestational age. When elevated above the level appropriate for gestational age, they may be associated with numerous other problems, including multiple gestations, threatened abortion, intrauterine demise, Rh disease, ectopic pregnancy, maternal or neonatal hepatitis, maternal hepatoma, gastrointestinal cancer, tumor metastatic to the liver, maternal herpes infection, fetal congenital cirrhosis, fetal tyrosinosis, preeclampsia, and fetal growth retardation. Other major malformations, such as omphalocele, nephrosis, or esophageal atresia, may also be associated. Levels of alpha-fetoprotein in amniotic fluid would be elevated in 90 percent of all infants with neural tube defects, but the concentration does not correlate with the severity of the disease. A fetus with a closed defect may not show an increased level of alpha-fetoprotein in the amniotic fluid, and elevated levels may return to normal at 24 weeks gestational age, even if a fetus does not have an open neural tube defect. However, amniocentesis combined with a detailed ultrasound evaluation of the fetal spine should accurately diagnose 95 to 99 percent of all cases.

37. DIAGNOSIS: CONTINUED CARE: ANSWER: E

(Sabiston and Spencer, 5/e, pp 1314-1331.) Ventricular septal defect accounts for 20 to 30 percent of all congenital cardiac anomalies. It may lead to cardiac failure and pulmonary hypertension if the defect is larger than 1 cm; or it may be asymptomatic if the defect is small. Surgery is not indicated for the asymptomatic patient with a small defect since a substantial number of these anomalies close spontaneously during the first few years of life. Operation is indicated in infants with congestive heart failure or rising pulmonary vascular resistance (owing to the left-to-right shunt). When symptoms are mild and can be controlled medically, operation is usually delayed until age 4 to 6. Operative mortality ranges from less than 5 percent to more than 20 percent depending on the degree of pulmonary vascular resistance.

38. HISTORY AND PHYSICAL: INITIAL WORKUP: ANSWER: A
(Isselbacher, 13/e, chap 26.) Bilateral conjugate eye movement to the side of the caloric stimulation indicates integrity of the brainstem pathways from the medulla to the midbrain (where the third nerve originates), as do full conjugate oculocephalic motions (doll's eye maneuvers). The absence of the rapid corrective phase manifested by nystagmus-like leftward eye gazing indicates a bilateral hemispheric lesion. Failure of an eye to adduct properly in the initial phase of the caloric response indicates a lesion in the ipsilateral third nerve (midbrain) or in the medial longitudinal fasciculus producing an internuclear ophthalmoplegia. In the former case, the pupil would be dilated and the eye abducted at rest.

39. HISTORY AND PHYSICAL: INITIAL WORKUP: ANSWER: C
(Isselbacher, 13/e, chap 375.) Very few diseases cause rapid dementia, noticeable in a period of weeks. Among them are depression, metabolic encephalopathy, encephalitis, poisoning, Binswanger's disease (white-matter infarction), and Creutzfeldt-Jakob disease. (Alzheimer's disease has a more insidious onset.) Creutzfeldt-Jakob disease is a slow-virus infection that causes a spongiform change in the cerebral cortex; it is characterized by rapid dementia, startle myoclonus, and, frequently, signs of occipital and cerebellar disease. CT scan and cerebrospinal fluid examination are nearly always normal in affected persons; after a period of time electroencephalography shows rapid, synchronous sharp waves, a diagnostic finding.

40. HISTORY AND PHYSICAL: INITIAL WORKUP: ANSWER: C
(Isselbacher, 13/e, chap 373.) Optic neuritis is the initial symptom in approximately 40 percent of persons who eventually are diagnosed as having multiple sclerosis. This rapidly developing ophthalmologic disorder is associated with partial or total loss of vision, pain on motion of the involved eye, scotoma affecting macular vision, and a variety of other visual-field defects. Ophthalmoscopically visible optic papillitis occurs in about half of cases.

41. PROGNOSIS: INITIAL WORKUP: ANSWER: E
(Isselbacher, 13/e, pp 2287-2291.) Multiple sclerosis is rare in non-temperate climates and common in western Europe and the United States. Both optic neuritis and internuclear ophthalmoplegia are common in multiple sclerosis and cause visual blurring. Prognosis is better in early adult onset multiple sclerosis than late adult onset disease. The findings in Choice D are rare in multiple sclerosis, as are isolated dementia, Parkinson-type syndromes, and aphasia. Magnetic resonance imaging of the brain is extremely sensitive for the demyelinating lesions of multiple sclerosis and is far superior to CT scan in the diagnosis and follow-up of multiple sclerosis patients.

42. DIAGNOSIS: INITIAL WORKUP: ANSWER: B
(Sabiston and Spencer, 5/e, pp 1314-1331.) Tetralogy of Fallot, transposition, and tricuspid atresia are cyanotic lesions. Congenital cyanosis that persists beyond the age of 2 years is associated, in the vast majority of cases, with a tetralogy of Fallot. Patent ductus arteriosus is associated with the characteristic continuous machinery murmur.

43. CLINICAL THERAPEUTICS: INITIAL WORKUP: ANSWER: B
(Isselbacher, 13/e, chaps 14, 380.) A disease of middle-aged and elderly patients, particularly women, paroxysmal facial pain (tic douloureux, trigeminal neuralgia) is usually of idiopathic origin. It may occur in association with multiple sclerosis, herpes zoster, or a tumor. Brief, intense, lancinating pains brought on by manipulation of trigger zones in the lips or face, without motor or sensory paralysis, characterize this disorder. The treatment of first choice is the anticonvulsant carbamazepine, which is effective in most patients. In cases of nonresponse or intolerance to carbamazepine, radiofrequency ablation of the gasserian ganglion of the trigeminal nerve may be beneficial.

44. DIAGNOSIS: EMERGENCY: ANSWER: E
(Droegemueller, pp 406-439.) In the management of ectopic pregnancies, clinical determination of serum hCG is important. The hCG doubling time ranges from 1.5 to 3.5 days. A discriminatory hCG zone is reached at 6500 mIU/mL. At this point, a gestational sac should be visualized in the uterus with transabdominal ultrasound. Transvaginal ultrasonography, however, has much higher resolution and can visualize an intrauterine gestational sac when hCG levels are around 2000 mIU/mL. Serum progesterone levels may be predictive of an abnormal pregnancy, but are not useful in the management of a patient in an emergency department setting. A culdocentesis would only be performed in a patient judged clinically unstable and in whom a hemoperitoneum was strongly suspected.

45. DIAGNOSTIC STUDIES: EMERGENCY: ANSWER: B
(Isselbacher, 13/e, chap 368.) The clinical picture presented in the question suggests acute subarachnoid hemorrhage, either from a ruptured saccular aneurysm or from an arteriovenous malformation. A CT scan of the head, done initially without infusion of contrast material, would be more likely than the other procedures listed to demonstrate the presence of blood in the subarachnoid space and possibly in the ventricles as well. In addition, a CT scan also can detect the presence of hydrocephalus and intracerebral hematoma, two conditions that, in the presence of coma, may require surgical intervention. Skull films are not likely to be informative in this case, although in the presence of a large arteriovenous malformation they may show intracranial calcification. Lumbar puncture as a means of establishing the presence of intracranial bleeding is rendered less useful and is possibly dangerous in this instance by the finding of retinal hemorrhages, a sign of acute intracranial hemorrhage. A radionuclide scan would have little to offer in this set of circumstances, and angiography would be premature.

46. CLINICAL INTERVENTION: EMERGENCY: ANSWER: C
(Isselbacher, 13/e, chap 376.) Treatment of hypotension, control of the airway, and a search for lesions that raise intracranial pressure are the first priorities in managing persons with severe head trauma. Skull x-rays have been largely replaced by CT scans because contusions and hemorrhages are better seen by CT scanning. Although stabilization of the neck is very important, the other treatment choices mentioned in the question are not.

47. DIAGNOSTIC STUDIES: CONTINUED CARE: ANSWER: E
(Isselbacher, 13/e, chap 39. Shiau, Ann Intern Med 102:773, 1985.) In the case described, the osmolality of fecal water is approximately equal to serum osmolality. Furthermore, there is no osmotic "gap" in the fecal water—the osmolality of the fecal water can be accounted for by the stool electrolyte composition: $[2 \times ([Na^+] + [K^+])] = [2 \times (39 + 96)] = 270$. A villous adenoma of the colon typically produces a secretory diarrhea. Lactose intolerance, nontropical sprue, and excessive use of milk of magnesia produce osmotic diarrheas with osmotic "gaps" caused by lactose, carbohydrates, and magnesium, respectively. Pancreatic insufficiency causes steatorrhea, not watery diarrhea.

48. HISTORY AND PHYSICAL: EMERGENCY: ANSWER: D
(Isselbacher, 13/e, chap 26.) In a comatose person, reactive pupils and the absence of eye movements in response to head turning or ice-water irrigation of the ear canals signify metabolic suppression of brainstem neurons. The major distinction that must be made is between true unresponsiveness and a "locked in" stroke state, in which eye movements also may be obliterated. In brain death, pupils are unreactive. A person unresponsive because of a conversion reaction cannot voluntarily suppress the nystagmus induced by caloric irrigation, although tonic eye movements can be suppressed by gaze fixation. Pontine hemorrhage is associated with small pupils. Bilateral infarcts in a carotid distribution may cause coma, but oculocephalic movements are normal.

49. CLINICAL THERAPEUTICS: CONTINUED CARE: ANSWER: E
(Berek, pp 441-449.) The condition of women who have hydatidiform moles but no evidence of metastatic disease should be followed routinely by hCG titers after uterine evacuation. Most authorities agree that prophylactic chemotherapy should not be employed in the routine management of women having hydatidiform moles because 85 to 90 percent of affected patients will require no further treatment. For a young woman in whom preservation of reproductive function is important, surgery is not routinely indicated.

50. DIAGNOSIS: EMERGENCY: ANSWER: D
(Youmans, 3/e, pp 1644-1689.) In the absence of trauma, a subarachnoid hemorrhage (SAH) is the most likely diagnosis. The most common cause of an SAH is a ruptured berry aneurysm (51 percent). Other less frequent causes include hypertensive hemorrhage, trauma, and bleeding from an arteriovenous malformation. The most characteristic symptom of an SAH is a sudden, severe headache. Associated with this symptom may be nausea and vomiting, neck stiffness, dizziness, photophobia, depressed consciousness, hypertension, and temperature elevation. The majority of intracranial aneurysms arise from the arteries composing the circle of Willis and at the origin of large vessels from the vertebrobasilar system. Roughly 40 percent of people with an aneurysmal SAH die before entering a hospital. Approximately 60 percent of those admitted recover to their premorbid state. Surgical clipping of the aneurysm neck is the standard treatment. Early surgical management of these patients (within 72 h of SAH) allows for prevention of aneurysmal rebleeding and aggressive management of posthemorrhage vasospasm.

51. CLINICAL THERAPEUTICS: CONTINUED CARE: ANSWER: C
(Isselbacher, 13/e, chap 356. Carmichael, Am J Med 76:1137, 1984. Ryan, Am J Med 77:501, 1984.) A direct effect of ingestion of aluminum in patients with renal failure is severe, unresponsive osteomalacia caused by its deposition at the site of osteoid mineralization. However, aluminum accumulation does not occur in patients with normal renal function, and the effects of long-term ingestion of aluminum hydroxide-containing antacids in such patients are a result of phosphorus depletion—that is, the binding of phosphorus by aluminum within the intestine prevents its absorption. In the absence of more specific symptoms, malnutrition is unlikely. Osteomalacia has been reported in association with benign tumors of mesenchymal origin (oncogenous osteomalacia) but not with gastric carcinomas.

52. CLINICAL INTERVENTION: CONTINUED CARE: ANSWER: A
(Nichols, pp 847-852.) In developing countries, obstetric injury remains the leading cause of vesicovaginal fistulas. In this country, vesicovaginal fistulas rarely occur after obstetric deliveries. Although fistulas can occur after radiation treatment, radical hysterectomy, or vaginal hysterectomy, they are three times more common with abdominal hysterectomy. It is thought that inadequate mobilization of the bladder or blunt dissection of the bladder from pubovesical fascia results in the formation of fistulas.

53. DIAGNOSTIC STUDIES: INITIAL WORKUP: ANSWER: E
(Isselbacher, 13/e, chap 340.) Low circulating levels of estrogens coupled with elevated gonadotropin levels exclude the presence of pituitary disease and indicate primary ovarian failure, which is premature at this patient's age. Bilateral tubal obstruction would cause infertility but not amenorrhea. Polycystic ovarian disease is associated with typical physical findings of weight gain and hirsutism, an earlier age of onset, and elevated circulating levels of estrogens. Exogenous administration of estrogens would lead to suppression of gonadotropin secretion.

54. DIAGNOSTIC STUDIES: CONTINUED CARE: ANSWER: C
(Isselbacher, 13/e, chaps 54, 144.) The differential diagnosis of grouped vesicular eruptions includes contact dermatitis and herpetic infections. Microscopic examination of the cellular material from the base of a fresh vesicle (less than 2 days old is best) stained with Giemsa reveals pathognomonic multinucleated giant cells diagnostic of a herpesvirus infection (varicella, zoster, or simplex). Unilateral dermatomal involvement establishes the diagnosis of shingles (herpes zoster). Neuralgia associated with zoster may precede the appearance of the cutaneous eruption and mimic myocardial infarction or acute cholecystitis.

55. CLINICAL THERAPEUTICS: CONTINUED CARE: ANSWER: E
(Isselbacher, 13/e, chap 144.) Herpes zoster will not respond to topical acyclovir. Oral or intravenous acyclovir may be helpful if dissemination occurs. Antibiotic therapy is indicated only for significant secondary bacterial infection. There is no evidence that fluorinated topical steroids are of help although systemic steroids are sometimes employed in the hope that the frequency of postherpetic neuralgia might be reduced. Most patients will respond to conservative therapy, which should include adequate oral pain medication and topical wet-to-dry saline or aluminum acetate (Domeboro) soaks to help dry up the vesicles and reduce the likelihood of secondary bacterial infection.

56. CLINICAL INTERVENTION: CONTINUED CARE: ANSWER: E
(Isselbacher, 13/e, chap 357.) Patients with primary hyperparathyroidism are usually asymptomatic, and mild degrees of hypercalcemia in such patients can usually be managed with adequate hydration. Whether observation alone is appropriate in these patients is controversial, especially when the diagnosis is made at a young age, since surveillance of renal function and bone status is lifelong and cumbersome. On the other hand, definitive treatment is clearly indicated when complications arise. In this patient, hypercalcemia and nephrolithiasis constitute a clear-cut indication for surgical treatment of the hyperparathyroidism. An additional reason would be to prevent bone loss in this young woman that would place her at an increased risk for development of skeletal complications at a later time. Glucocorticoids are usually ineffective in the management of primary hyperparathyroidism and would affect bone metabolism negatively, besides producing other serious side effects when administered on a long-term basis. Thiazide diuretics or calcium supplementation are contraindicated in this patient because of the risk of inducing hypercalcemia.

57. CLINICAL INTERVENTION: CONTINUED CARE: ANSWER: E

(Isselbacher, 13/e, chaps 356, 357.) The hypercalcemia of sarcoidosis is usually associated with disseminated disease. Therefore, almost all persons with sarcoidosis who have hypercalcemia also have an abnormal chest x-ray (diffuse fibronodular infiltration or marked enlargement of hilar nodes, or both). This is an important point in the differential diagnosis of hypercalcemia—sarcoidosis is unlikely as a cause of hypercalcemia if the chest x-ray is normal. Hypergammaglobulinemia is another helpful clue to the presence of sarcoidosis. The hypercalcemia of sarcoidosis is thought to be the consequence of increased synthesis of 1,25$(OH)_2$ vitamin D_3 and the subsequent increased intestinal absorption of calcium. Elevated serum calcium concentration in sarcoidosis causes a decreased level of serum parathyroid hormone, resulting in marked hypercalciuria.

58. HISTORY AND PHYSICAL: CONTINUED CARE: ANSWER: C

(DiSaia, 4/e, pp 158-161.) Postmenopausal bleeding is the most common presenting symptom of women who have endometrial carcinoma. Because this warning signal is present even in the earliest stage of the disease, early diagnosis and treatment are possible. In fact, approximately 70 percent of affected women have stage I disease when they first seek treatment.

59. DIAGNOSTIC STUDIES: CONTINUED CARE: ANSWER: D

(Isselbacher, 13/e, chap 340.) Asherman's syndrome, destruction of the endometrium, occurs after vigorous curettage, usually in association with postpartum hemorrhage or therapeutic abortion. The diagnosis is confirmed by hysterosalpingography or by direct visualization of the scarred endometrium using a hysteroscope. Treatment consists of dilation and curettage, followed by the insertion of an intrauterine device for 8 weeks.

60. CLINICAL INTERVENTION: CONTINUED CARE: ANSWER: A

(Isselbacher, 13/e, pp 1265-1266.) Only 50 percent of patients with acute renal failure will be oliguric (urine output of 400 mL/d or less). The *sin qua non* of acute renal failure is a rapid decrease in glomerular filtration rate and subsequent retention of nitrogenous wastes. It is frequently asymptomatic and not necessarily associated with uremic symptoms. Only 40 percent of cases of acute renal failure are due to intrinsic renal causes. The majority are prerenal (renal hypoperfusion states) or postrenal (obstructive uropathy), and most cases are reversible.

61. HEALTH MAINTENANCE: CONTINUED CARE: ANSWER: A

(Schwartz, 6/e, pp 637-639.) There is an unusually high incidence of carcinoma of the nasopharynx among Chinese. In the early stages of the disease, metastases remain confined to the neck. Diagnosis of nasopharyngeal cancer, which tends to arise in relatively young people, should be made by biopsy of the primary tumor. Biopsy of the neck nodes should be avoided because implantation of the tumor in skin and subcutaneous tissue may occur. Radiation therapy is the treatment of choice for the primary nasopharyngeal cancer. Cervical metastases that remain clinically evident should be removed by a radical neck dissection.

62. CLINICAL INTERVENTION: INITIAL WORKUP: ANSWER: D
(Schwartz, 6/e, pp 1078-1079.) Premature contraction of the cricopharyngeus muscle on swallowing, which leads to partial obstruction, is believed to be the cause of this diverticulum of the pharyngoesophageal junction. High intraluminal pressure results in an outpouching of mucosa through the oblique fibers of the pharyngeal constrictors. Dysphagia is common and is the usual presenting symptom. The diagnosis is established by barium swallow. Treatment is surgical: diverticulectomy or suspension of the diverticulum is usually recommended. Because the diverticulum is located above the superior esophageal sphincter, no mechanism exists to prevent aspiration of the contents of the diverticulum. Pulmonary complications are common.

63. HISTORY AND PHYSICAL: CONTINUED CARE: ANSWER: E
(Isselbacher, 13/e, pp 1358-1359.) Long-standing gastroesophageal reflux can induce fibrotic strictures as a result of chronic reflux esophagitis. These strictures are typically fibrotic and short (1-3 cm). They occur just above the lower esophageal sphincter. A second form of stricture also can occur in the setting of long-standing reflux. The esophageal mucosa undergoes metaplasia and islands, or tongues, of columnar epithelium extend proximally from the EG junction into the mid or upper esophagus. This is termed Barrett's esophagitis and can cause proximal esophageal strictures. Of more concern is the increased incidence of adenocarcinoma in these areas of metaplasia, occurring in up to 5 percent of patients with Barrett's esophagitis. All three strictures can result in food sticking in the esophagus. Simple esophagitis may cause pain and bleeding but, unless complicated by a stricture, would not likely cause obstruction. Achalasia is unrelated to gastroesophageal reflux. It is due to incomplete relaxation of the lower esophageal sphincter which normally relaxes with swallowing. However, dysphagia, chest pain, and regurgitation are commom symptoms and so achalasia should be considered in this case.

64. DIAGNOSIS: CONTINUED CARE: ANSWER: D
(Isselbacher, 13/e, chaps 41, 268.) The x-ray presented in the question demonstrates esophageal varices, which are associated with portal hypertension. Of the diseases listed, only Laënnec's cirrhosis would lead directly to portal hypertension. Although the other lesions might be associated with upper gastrointestinal bleeding, none would be expected to produce varices.

65. HEALTH MAINTENANCE: CONTINUED CARE: ANSWER: D
(Remington, 3/e, pp 306-320.) Current data indicate that most pediatric cases of HIV and AIDS infections are acquired perinatally from infected women. Transmissions may occur during pregnancy, during labor and delivery, or in the immediate postpartum period. AIDS has also been reported in children delivered of HIV-positive mothers who underwent cesarean section. Therefore, no apparent protection is offered by this mode of delivery. Cesarean section should be reserved for obstetric indication only. The rate of perinatal transmission varies widely between studies, but it is probably high (as high as 65 percent in one study). However, the transmission of disease from an infected mother to her infant is not absolute, as evidenced by healthy HIV-negative infants delivered to HIV-positive mothers. The current recommendation is that infected mothers be advised to postpone pregnancy until further studies are done and more definite information can be obtained. HIV has been isolated from breast milk of infected mothers and for this reason these mothers should be advised against breastfeeding to avoid any postnatal transmission.

66. HEALTH MAINTENANCE: CONTINUED CARE: ANSWER: D

(Isselbacher, 13/e, pp 1480-1481.) Progression to cirrhosis occurs in 20 to 50 percent of patients with chronic HCV, even in patients without symptoms and with only modest transaminase elevations. Liver biopsy abnormalities will be demonstated in up to 50 percent of the cases despite normal transaminase levels in asymptomatic carriers. Glucocorticoids are not effective in treating chronic HCV. Interferon has been shown to be effective with lower transaminase levels and HCV RNA may become undetectable with this therapy. This finding does not preclude relapse, however. Following hepatic transplantation, reinfection with HCV is nearly universal though allographic failure due to recurrent infection is quite rare.

67. CLINICAL THERAPEUTICS: CONTINUED CARE: ANSWER: C

(Isselbacher, 13/e, chap 252.) The causes of stomal (anastomotic) ulceration following peptic ulcer surgery include incomplete vagotomy, retained gastric antrum, the Zollinger-Ellison syndrome (gastrinoma), poor gastric emptying, and ingestion of ulcerogenic drugs. In the case presented, if the previous antrectomy had been complete, the serum gastrin level should not be elevated. An elevated serum gastrin level that declines after intravenous administration of secretin is characteristic of a retained gastric antrum attached to the duodenal stump. Neither frequent antacid therapy nor a total vagotomy is effective in healing a stomal ulcer; thus, resection of the retained antrum is indicated. In the Zollinger-Ellison syndrome, the serum gastrin level paradoxically increases after intravenous infusion of secretin.

68. CLINICAL THERAPEUTICS: CONTINUED CARE: ANSWER: A

(Evans, pp 95-98. Herbst, 2/e, p 295.) All spermicides contain an ingredient, usually nonoxynol 9, that immobilizes or kills sperm on contact. They provide a mechanical barrier and need to be placed into the vagina before each coital act. Their effectiveness increases with increasing age of the women who use them—probably due to increased motivation. The effectiveness is similar to that of the diaphragm. Although it has been reported that contraceptive failures with spermicides may be associated with an increased incidence of congenital malformations, this finding has not been confirmed in several large studies and is not believed to be valid.

69. PROGNOSIS: CONTINUED CARE: ANSWER: E

(Isselbacher, 13/e, p 1419.) Meckel's diverticulum is a common congenital anomaly of the GI tract affecting 2 percent of all patients at autopsy. The diverticulum occurs along the antimesenteric of the small bowel within 100 cm of the ileocecal valve. The presence of ectopic gastric mucosa within the Meckel's diverticulum can lead to ulceration of and bleeding from the adjacent bowel. This ectopic gastric mucosa can be detected during a nuclear medicine scan utilizing sodium pertechnatate. In a child with intussusception in which a lead point is discovered, the most frequent cause of the condition is Meckel's diverticulum. There is no malignant potential reported with Meckel's diverticulum.

70. PROGNOSIS: INITIAL WORKUP: ANSWER: D

(Isselbacher, 13/e, pp 1427-1429.) Adenocarcinoma of the colon limited to the mucosa and submucosa is Dukes stage A and has a greater than 90 percent 5-year survival rate. Invasion of the entire thickness of the colonic wall (stage B2) and regional lymph nodes (stage C) reduces the 5-year survival to 70 to 85 percent and 30 to 60 percent respectively. The presence of elevated carcinoembryonic antigen (CEA) preoperatively, even in the absence of demonstrable metastases, is suggestive of eventual recurrence and is a poor prognostic indicator. Recurrences are uncommon at the surgical anastomotic site if the margins are initially free of tumor. The lifetime risk of a second carcinoma occurring, metachronous lesion, is 3 to 5 percent with the risk of subsequent adenomatous polyps developing in 15 percent of patients.

71. DIAGNOSIS: CONTINUED CARE: ANSWER: C

(Wilmore, vol 2, sect 9, chap 1, pp 33-35.) An immunocompromised host may not manifest some of the more typical signs and symptoms of infection, such as elevated temperature and white count; this forces the clinician to focus on more subtle signs and symptoms. Early sepsis is a physiologically hyperdynamic, hypermetabolic state representing a surge of catecholamines, cortisol, and other stress-related hormones. A changing mental status, tachypnea that leads to respiratory alkalosis, and flushed skin are often the earliest manifestations of sepsis. Intermittent hypotension requiring increased fluid resuscitation to maintain adequate urine output is characteristic of occult sepsis. Hyperglycemia and insulin resistance during sepsis are typical in diabetic as well as nondiabetic patients. This relates to the gluconeogenic state of the stress response. The cardiovascular response to early sepsis is characterized by an increased cardiac output, decreased systemic vascular resistance, and decreased peripheral utilization of oxygen, which yields a decreased arteriovenous oxygen difference.

72. CLINICAL THERAPEUTICS: CONTINUED CARE: ANSWER: B

(Schwartz, 6/e, p 113.) Administration of lactated Ringer's solution is appropriate for replacing gastrointestinal losses and correcting extracellular fluid deficits. Containing 130 meq/L sodium, lactated Ringer's is hypoosmolar with respect to sodium and provides approximately 150 mL of free water with each liter given. Although ordinarily not a significant load, in some clinical situations it can be. Lactated Ringer's is sufficiently "physiological" to enable administration of large amounts without affecting the body's acid-base balance significantly.

73. DIAGNOSIS: CONTINUED CARE: ANSWER: C

(Isselbacher, 13/e, chap 268.) Persons who have cirrhosis, particularly alcoholic cirrhosis and ascites, may develop acute bacterial peritonitis without a clearly definable precipitating event. The clinical presentation of spontaneous bacterial peritonitis may be subtle, such as fever of unknown origin and mild abdominal pain, and be attributed to other causes. Diagnosis is based on a careful examination of ascitic fluid obtained by paracentesis and should include cell count, Gram's stain, and culture.

74. HEALTH MAINTENANCE: CONTINUED CARE: ANSWER: E

(Isselbacher, 13/e, pp 1521-1527.) Acute pancreatitis most often is due to gallstone passage or alcoholism. Most cases are self-limited and resolve with sequelae. 10 percent of patients will develop a pancreatic abscess and 15 percent will develop pancreatic pseudocysts. Both clinical (Ranson/Imrie) and CT indices have been proposed to grade the severity of acute pancreatitis. The presence of three or more Ranson factors, and/or a CT severity score of greater than 7 are poor prognostic factors. When clinical findings put the patient in the high risk group, three or more Ranson factors are present, AND there is suspicion for gallstone pancreatitis, ERCP should be performed urgently.

75. CLINICAL INTERVENTION: CONTINUED CARE: ANSWER: B

(Reece, pp 908-909, 1061-1062.) The incidence of appendicitis in pregnancy is 1:2000, unchanged from that of the nonpregnant population. The diagnosis is very difficult in pregnancy. Leukocytosis, nausea, and vomiting are common in pregnancy. The upward displacement of the appendix by the uterus may cause appendicitis to simulate cholecystitis, pyelonephritis, gastritis, or degenerating myomata. Surgery is necessary even if the diagnosis is not certain. Delays in surgery due to difficulty in diagnosis as the appendix moves up are probably the cause of an increasing maternal mortality with increasing gestational age. Premature birth and abortion account for a rate of fetal loss close to 15 percent.

76. HEALTH MAINTENANCE: INITIAL WORKUP: ANSWER: B

(Isselbacher, 13/e, chap 258.) Carcinoma of the colon is the most common cause of mechanical obstruction of the colon and is followed in frequency by sigmoid diverticulitis and volvulus. These three causes account for 90 percent of cases of colonic obstruction. Adhesions and hernias cause about 75 percent of cases of small-intestine obstruction but are uncommon causes of colonic obstruction.

77. DIAGNOSTIC STUDIES: INITIAL WORKUP: ANSWER: D

(Isselbacher, 13/e, chap 255.) Radiographic demonstration of luminal narrowing, mucosal ulceration, and cobblestoning in the ileum is compatible with a diagnosis of regional enteritis. In Whipple's disease, x-rays characteristically show marked thickening of mucosal folds in the duodenum and jejunum. On barium enema, an appendiceal abscess usually presents as a mass indenting the cecal tip. Adenocarcinoma of the small bowel usually occurs as an ulcerated mass lesion in the duodenum. Infiltrating lymphomas of the distal bowel may be difficult to distinguish from regional enteritis radiographically, but stenotic bowel segments would not suggest lymphoma.

78. CLINICAL THERAPEUTICS: CONTINUED CARE: ANSWER: C

(Isselbacher, 13/e, chap 255.) Sigmoidoscopic demonstration of a hyperemic mucosa studded with plaquelike lesions is characteristic of pseudomembranous (antibiotic-associated) colitis, which is caused by the enterotoxin of *Clostridium difficile*. Although symptoms commonly develop while the offending antibiotic is still being taken, the syndrome may not become evident until several days or weeks after completion of therapy. Ischemic colitis may cause bloody diarrhea but not the mucosal lesions described. Amebic or *Shigella* infestation is associated with punched-out ulcerations of the mucosa. Toxic megacolon is a complication of active colitis. Treatment is directed at either binding the toxin (cholestyramine) or eradicating the bacteria (oral vancomycin or metronidazole).

79. HEALTH MAINTENANCE: CONTINUED CARE: ANSWER: D

(Evans, pp 6-10.) The risk of aneuploidy is increased with multiple miscarriages not attributable to other causes such as endocrine abnormalities or cervical incompetence. Paternal age does not contribute significantly to aneuploidy until probably age 55, and most risks of paternal age are for point mutations. A 45,X karyotype results from loss of chromosome material and does not have increased risks for nondisjunctional errors. Similarly, induced ovulation does not result in increased nondisjunction.

80. HISTORY AND PHYSICAL: INITIAL WORKUP: ANSWER: A
(Isselbacher, 13/e, chap 311.) Hodgkin's disease can be distinguished from non-Hodgkin's lymphomas (NHL) by a variety of characteristics. The "B" (or constitutional) symptoms described for Hodgkin's disease are less common in patients with NHL, although the presence of these symptoms is thought to influence the prognosis negatively. Involvement of Waldeyer's ring occurs more commonly in NHL than in Hodgkin's disease. Extralymphatic presentation is more frequent with NHL than with Hodgkin's disease, and NHL is more often disseminated at the time of diagnosis. Approximately 60 percent of all lymphomas are NHL.

81. PROGNOSIS: CONTINUED CARE: ANSWER: C
(Isselbacher, 13/e, chaps 317, 322.) Ninety percent of persons with nonseminomatous germ cell tumors produce either α-fetoprotein (AFP) or β-hCG; in contrast, persons with pure seminomas usually produce neither. These tumor markers are present for some time after surgery—if the presurgical levels are high, 30 days or more may be required before meaningful postsurgical levels can be obtained. The half-lives of AFP and β-hCG are 6 days and 1 day, respectively. After treatment, unequal reduction of β-hCG and AFP may occur, suggesting that the two markers are synthesized by heterogeneous clones of cells within the tumor; thus, both markers should be followed. β-hCG is similar to luteinizing hormone except for its distinctive beta subunit.

82. CLINICAL INTERVENTION: INITIAL WORKUP: ANSWER: D
(Isselbacher, 13/e, chap 311.) Neoplasms may be classified as to their cell of origin by the use of antisera and monoclonal antibodies against certain cell surface phenotypic markers and, more recently, by the use of DNA probes for immunoglobulin genes and genes for the beta chain of the T-cell receptor. The malignant cell in chronic lymphocytic leukemia is a morphologically normal but functionally abnormal B lymphocyte. Follicular lymphomas arise from the proliferative part of the B-cell system, the lymphoid follicle, while the diffuse, small lymphocytic lymphomas are derived from the secretory compartment of the medullary cords. The Burkitt's lymphoma cell is a malignant cell of B-lymphocyte lineage; in many cases it bears a characteristic chromosomal translocation. In contrast to these B-cell neoplasms, mycosis fungoides is a peripheral T-cell lymphoma in which helper-cell function and phenotype have been identified.

83. APPLYING BASIC CONCEPTS: CONTINUED CARE: ANSWER: A
(Verkauf, pp 207-217.) Failure of fusion of the müllerian ducts can give rise to the several types of uterine anomalies of which uterus bicornis unicollis is a representative type. This condition is associated with higher obstetric complications, such as an increase in the rate of second-trimester abortion and premature labor. If the pregnancies go to term, malpresentations such as breech and transverse lies are frequent. Also, prolonged labor, which is probably due to inadequate muscle development in the uterus, increased bleeding, and a higher incidence of fetal anomalies caused by defective implantation of the placenta all occur far more commonly than in normal pregnancies. An intravenous pyelogram is mandatory in the workup of patients with uterine anomalies as there is an associated higher incidence of urinary tract anomalies. In uterus bicornis unicollis, there is a single cervix with a normal vagina.

84. APPLYING BASIC CONCEPTS: CONTINUED CARE: ANSWER: C
(Isselbacher, 13/e, pp 1099-1100.) Chronic inflammation or fibrotic changes of the pericardium can lead to a constrictive pericarditis. The lack of distensibility of the thickened pericardium leads to impedence

of ventricular filling in late diastole and the square root configuration of the ventricular pressure curve. This latter finding is also found in restrictive cardiomyopathies and is not pathognomonic of constrictive pericarditis. This lack of distensibility of the pericardial sac also leads to equalization of the atrial pressures at an elevated level often greater than 15mmHg and a positive Kussmaul's sign. Kussmaul's sign refers to a rise in jugular venous pressure with inspiration. The pericardial thickening and calcification is demonstrable with CT scanning, especially electron beam scanners that can provide cardiac gating and true cine-CT of the heart.

85. HISTORY AND PHYSICAL: INITIAL WORKUP: ANSWER: D
(Isselbacher, 13/e, chap 195.) Many persons who have ankle edema are inappropriately diagnosed as having heart failure. In particular, the diagnosis of right heart failure should not be made in the absence of jugular venous distention. Venous varicosities, cyclic edema, thrombophlebitis, and hypoalbuminemia all cause ankle edema and should be considered in the differential diagnosis.

86. APPLYING BASIC CONCEPTS: EMERGENCY: ANSWER: D
(Schwartz, 6/e, p 491.) Central venous pressure can be affected by a variety of factors including those of cardiac, noncardiac, and artifactual origin. Venous tone, right ventricular compliance, intrathoracic pressure, and blood volume all influence central venous pressure. Vasoconstrictor drugs, positive pressure ventilation (with and without PEEP), mediastinal compression, and hypervolemia all increase central venous pressure.

87. CLINICAL INTERVENTION: CONTINUED CARE: ANSWER: D
(Schwartz, 6/e, pp 993-994.) The problem of deep vein thrombosis and pulmonary embolism is significant in general surgery. There are approximately 2.5 million episodes of deep vein thrombosis and 600,000 pulmonary embolic events that result in 200,000 deaths annually. The problem is exacerbated by the disorder's frequent unheralded progression—only 20 to 25 percent of fatal pulmonary emboli are suspected clinically by the physician or manifest by classic signs or symptoms. The fact that most deaths due to pulmonary embolism occur before effective therapy can be started highlights the importance of preventive measures. Several documented factors help identify those at increased risk, including age greater than 40, obesity, malignancy, venous disease, congestive heart failure and atrial fibrillation, and prolonged bed rest. Virchow initially attributed venous thrombosis to the combination of venous stasis, hypercoagulability, and endothelial injury. The first two conditions are exacerbated by operative positioning and stress such that 25 percent of patients at moderate risk will develop venous thromboembolism, 50 percent within 24 h and 80 percent within 72 h postoperatively. The recommendation for prophylaxis in those at high risk is preoperative anticoagulation with warfarin. No prophylaxis is recommended for those at low risk (e.g, those less than age 40 with normal weight and no venous disease). Prophylactic regimens for those at moderate risk are basically chemical or mechanical, and the best two, which have equivalent effec:iveness, are representative of each type. First, low-dose heparin (5000 units) started 2 h preoperatively and continued every 12 h postoperatively will decrease the risk of deep vein thrombosis from 25 to 7 percent and of major pulmonary embolus from 6 to 0.6 percent. External pneumatic compression devices not only obviate venous stasis, but they also have a systemic effect on coagulation, such that use on the arms also significantly reduces venous thromboembolism of the lower extremities. Early ambulation, elastic stockings, leg elevation, and dipyridamole (Persantine) alone have not been documented to be effective.

88. CLINICAL INTERVENTION: EMERGENCY: ANSWER: C

(Isselbacher, 13/e, p 1076.) Right ventricular infarctions rarely occur in isolation but biventricular necrosis following a myocardial infarction involving the inferoposterior MI is common. The hemodynamic findings are similar to constrictive pericarditis or tamponade. The elevated central venous pressure secondary to right ventricular myocardial damage is manifested by elevated jugular venous pressure, hepatomegaly, and hypotension. Volume therapy will often be successful in correcting hypotension and low right ventricular output which can complicate extensive right ventricular infarction.

89. CLINICAL THERAPEUTICS: EMERGENCY: ANSWER: D

(Isselbacher, 13/e, chap 203. Muller, Ann Intern Med 108:1, 1988. TIMI Study Group, N Engl J Med 320:618, 1989.) The sooner thrombolytic therapy is started after the onset of symptoms, the greater the likelihood of benefit. Patients treated within 1 to 3 h will benefit most. Though tPA is more effective than streptokinase in restoring patency of vessels, a difference in mortality has not been demonstrated. Although the optimum adjunctive anticoagulant and antiplatelet regimen has not yet been established, up to 325 mg of aspirin and 5000 units of heparin should be given on the day of treatment and continued for up to 5 days. Any evidence for reocclusion, such as recurrent chest pain or ST elevation, should be met with emergent angioplasty, readministration of thrombolytic therapy, or surgical revascularization, depending on circumstances.

90. CLINICAL INTERVENTION: CONTINUED CARE: ANSWER: B

(Isselbacher, 13/e, p 1098.) The patient's history of chest trauma associated with fever and a friction rub strongly suggests a postcardiac injury syndrome. This syndrome can follow myocardial contusion, infarction, or penetrating trauma. Symptoms typically occur within one month of the initial insult and last for approximately one week, but tend to recur over several months to years. Symptomatic treatment with aspirin is usually sufficient. The occurrence of pericardial effusion is quite rare. The exact etiology of this syndrome is not clear but may relate to a hypersensitivity reaction to an antigen released or formed following the cardiac injury. Viral infection also may play a role.

91. DIAGNOSTIC STUDIES: INITIAL WORKUP: ANSWER: E

(Isselbacher, 13/e, chap 282.) Urticaria and angioedema are common disorders, affecting approximately 20 percent of the population. In acute urticarial angioedema, attacks of swelling are of less than 6 weeks' duration; chronic urticarial angioedema is by definition more longstanding. Urticaria usually is pruritic and affects the trunk and proximal extremities. Angioedema is generally less pruritic and affects the hands, feet, genitalia, and face. The woman described in the question has chronic urticaria, which probably is due to a cutaneous necrotizing vasculitis. The clues to the diagnosis are the arthralgias, presence of residual skin discoloration, and elevated sedimentation rate—these would be uncharacteristic of other urticarial diseases. Diagnosis can be confirmed by skin biopsy. Chronic urticaria is rarely of allergic cause; hence, allergy skin tests and measurement of total immunoglobulin E levels are not helpful. Measurement of C1 esterase inhibitor activity is useful in diagnosing hereditary angioedema, a disease not associated with urticaria. Patch tests are used to diagnose contact dermatitis.

92. DIAGNOSIS: CONTINUED CARE: ANSWER: D

(Isselbacher, 13/e, chap 291.) Polyarteritis nodosa is a vasculitis of medium-sized vessels. Early systemic features include fever, weakness, anorexia, weight loss, myalgias, and arthralgias (though severe and persistent arthritis is uncommon). Pericarditis and pleuritis also can occur. Mononeuritis multiplex develops because of involvement of the vasa nervorum; it is reflected in the man described by

the sudden loss of the ability to dorsiflex his right great toe. Abdominal pain occurs in 60 to 70 percent of affected persons and is related to disease involvement of mesenteric arteries. Hypertension develops from arterial occlusion and occurs before renal involvement. Laboratory findings of elevated erythrocyte sedimentation rate, anemia of chronic disease, and polymorphonuclear leukocytosis all occur with polyarteritis nodosa. Pulmonary involvement is unusual and serves to distinguish this entity clinically from allergic granulomatosis and Wegener's granulomatosis. Hypersensitivity vasculitis is a term applied to small-vessel vasculitides associated with a range of findings—from purely cutaneous disease to minimal skin disease but life-threatening involvement of major organs. Giant cell arteritis involves the aorta and other great vessels, producing constitutional symptoms and large-vessel occlusion in young women (Takayasu's disease) and in the elderly (temporal arteritis, polymyalgia rheumatica).

93. CLINICAL INTERVENTION: CONTINUED CARE: ANSWER: D
(Isselbacher, 13/e, pp 1621-1623.) Multiple myeloma nearly always is associated with M paraproteinuria; its absence suggests light chain disease. Half of multiple myeloma patients will have renal damage but only 25 percent will develop renal failure during the course of the disease. Renal damage is multifactorial and may be tubular or glomerular in origin. Because of the increased protein in the serum, hyperviscosity develops which occurs at lower concentrations of paraproteinemia with IgM rather than IgG or IgA. Benign monoclonal gammopathy is much more common than multiple myeloma and can be distinguished from it by the lack of anemia and hypercalcemia, absence of urinary Bence Jones protein, greater than 5 percent marrow plasmacytosis, and a labeling index of less than 1 percent. Extramedullary lymphoid tissue is not typically involved with the plasmacytosis associated with multiple myeloma and thus splenomegaly and lymphadenopathy are unusual.

94. DIAGNOSIS: INITIAL WORKUP: ANSWER: D
(Schwartz, 6/e, pp 1574-1576.) Clinical manifestations of adrenocortical insufficiency include hyperkalemia, hyponatremia, hypoglycemia, fever, weight loss, and dehydration. There is excessive sodium loss in the urine, contraction of the plasma volume, and perhaps hypotension or shock. Classic hyperpigmentation is present in *chronic* Addison's disease only. Addison's disease may present in newborns as a congenital atrophy, as an insidious chronic state often due to tuberculosis, as an acute dysfunction secondary to trauma or adrenal hemorrhage, or as a semiacute adrenal insufficiency seen during stress or surgery. In this last instance, signs and symptoms include nausea, lassitude, vomiting, fever, progressive salt wasting, hyperkalemia, and hypoglycemia. It may be confirmed by measurements of urinary Na^+ loss and absence of response to ACTH.

95. APPLYING BASIC CONCEPTS: CONTINUED CARE: ANSWER: E
(Isselbacher, 13/e, chap 280.) Plasma cell diseases are a group of conditions in which a clone of cells capable of synthesizing and secreting immunoglobulins, or the heavy or light chain component of these molecules, proliferates abnormally. IgG immunoglobulins are the most common class produced in such diseases. Also, free light chains usually are produced in excess and are detected in urine as Bence Jones protein. Multiple myeloma is the most common plasma cell neoplasm. Its classic presentation includes bone pain, anemia, hypercalcemia, renal failure, and recurrent infections in an elderly person. Diagnosis is best made by looking for a homogeneous globulin peak on electrophoresis of serum, urine, or both. Waldenström's macroglobulinemia is a related condition in which the monoclonal immunoglobulin is of the IgM class. Because IgM is so large (it circulates as a pentamer), it is restricted to the bloodstream and in high concentrations tends to cause hyperviscosity of the blood. Other features differentiating Waldenström's macroglobulinemia from multiple myeloma are enlargement of lymph nodes and spleen and occasional transformation to chronic lymphocytic leukemia or lymphocytic lymphoma.

96. APPLYING BASIC CONCEPTS: INITIAL WORKUP: ANSWER: E
(Becker, p 944.) Delayed puberty in general is defined as absent breast budding by age 13 and delay in progression is defined as the elapsing of 5 years between onset of breast changes and the expected menarche. There are five etiologic classifications of delayed puberty. The first is constitutional delay, which is more common in girls than boys and runs in families. The second is hypergonadotropic hypogonadism, of which gonadal dysgenesis is an example. Patients with Turner syndrome are in this category. Another class is hypogonadotropic hypogonadism, which includes CNS diseases such as tumors or meningoencephalitis. The fourth class is gonadotropin deficiency, such as is seen in patients with anorexia and others with pituitary deficiency. Lastly, there is normogonadotropic hypogonadism, as in end-organ defects such as müllerian agenesis and testicular feminization.

97. HISTORY AND PHYSICAL: CONTINUED CARE: ANSWER: B
(Gomel, pp 164-165.) Describing an obstetric history by the four-digit system is more comprehensive than merely indicating gravidity and parity. The first digit of the four indicates the number of term infants delivered; the second, the number of premature infants delivered; the third, the number of abortions; and the fourth, the number of children now alive. A woman described as 7-2-1-6, therefore, has had seven term deliveries, two premature deliveries, and one abortion; six of her children currently are alive.

98. APPLYING BASIC CONCEPTS: INITIAL WORKUP: ANSWER: A
(Schwartz, 5/e, pp 1215-1216.) Blind loop syndrome occurs as a result of bacterial overgrowth in a stagnant portion of the small intestine. Stricture, stenosis, diverticula, and blind pouches predispose to this condition. Intestinal obstruction is not typically present. Bacteria compete successfully for vitamin B_{12}, causing megaloblastic anemia not responsive to intrinsic factor therapy. Steatorrhea occurs from deconjugation of bile salts by bacteria. Palliative treatment consists of oral tetracycline and B_{12}; however, recalcitrant symptoms should be treated by surgical correction of the blind loop.

99. HEALTH MAINTENANCE: CONTINUED CARE: ANSWER: A
(Isselbacher, 13/e, chap 289.) The diagnosis of ankylosing spondylitis is made on clinical grounds. Historical features suggesting inflammatory back disease include pain and prolonged stiffness that are worse at night and during rest periods and characteristically relieved with activity. In contrast, mechanical low back pain usually is eased with bed rest and made worse with activity, such as sitting, standing, walking, and lifting. Signs of nerve-root compression are not part of the clinical spectrum of ankylosing spondylitis. Ankylosing spondylitis usually presents before the age of 40 years; on the other hand, degenerative joint disease and degenerative disk disease are common causes of back pain in the elderly. Back pain made worse with walking and improved with rest and lumbar flexion is characteristic of the pseudoclaudication syndrome associated with lumbar spinal stenosis.

100. LEGAL AND ETHICAL ISSUES: INITIAL WORKUP: ANSWER: B
(Herbst, 2/e, pp 363-368, 373-375.) Sexual assault happens to people of all ages. The mentally and physically handicapped and the very old are particularly susceptible. Victims of rape should always be treated as victims and at no time should the implication of guilt be applied to them. Psychologic reaction to rape includes two phases: an immediate phase of paralysis of the coping mechanisms, usually lasting hours or days, followed by a more prolonged period of reorganization that may last months to years. The victim's menstrual history, birth control regimen, and known pregnancy status should be assessed at the initial examination. In the experience of most sexual assault centers, the chance that pregnancy will occur

as a result of sexual assault is quite small and has been estimated to be approximately 2 to 4 percent for victims having a single, unprotected coitus. If the patient has been exposed at midcycle, the risk would obviously be higher. "Morning after" prophylaxis by high-dose estrogens or oral contraceptives should be offered to unprotected rape victims. About 10 percent of all abused children are also sexually abused. Although the crime is underreported, it is estimated that about 336,000 children are sexually abused each year in the United States. Incestual activity may be experienced by as many as 15 to 25 percent of women and 12 percent of men. A family member is the sexual abuser of a child in about 80 percent of cases. Father-daughter incest accounts for about 75 percent of reported cases. A brother-sister relationship may be the most common type of incest but is reported less frequently.

101. APPLYING BASIC CONCEPTS: INITIAL WORKUP: ANSWER: D
(Schwartz, 5/e, p 1212.) Meckel's diverticulum is found on the antimesenteric border of the ileum within the first 3 feet of the ileocecal valve. It may contain gastric mucosa and peptic ulceration may lead to bleeding. However, the most common complication in affected adults is obstruction. This may result from volvulus of a portion of intestine around a band that can sometimes be seen extending from the tip of the diverticulum to the umbilicus or abdominal wall. Obstruction may be due to intussusception, with the diverticulum as the lead point.

102. DIAGNOSIS: INITIAL WORKUP: ANSWER: E
(Rudolph, 19/e, pp 1871-1876.) In infants, achromic skin patches, especially in association with infantile spasms, are characteristic of tuberous sclerosis. Other dermal abnormalities (adenoma sebaceum and subungual fibromata) associated with this disorder appear later in childhood. Although children who have neurofibromatosis may have a few achromic patches, the identifying dermal lesions are café au lait spots. Incontinentia pigmenti also is associated with seizures; the skin lesions typical of this disorder begin as bullous eruptions that later become hyperpigmented lesions. Pityriasis rosea and psoriasis are not associated with infantile spasms.

103. CLINICAL INTERVENTION: CONTINUED CARE: ANSWER: C
(Isselbacher, 13/e, chap 284. Balow, Ann Intern Med 106:79, 1987.) Renal disease is clinically evident in about half those persons with systemic lupus erythematosus (SLE). However, nearly all persons with SLE have some evidence of renal disease on renal biopsy. Renal disease associated with SLE includes both glomerulonephritis and interstitial nephritis. Glomerular disease has been classified into membranous nephritis and mesangial, focal, and diffuse glomerulonephritis. Immune-complex interstitial nephritis occurs most commonly in persons who have diffuse glomerulonephritis. Urinalysis performed for persons with active renal disease usually reveals microscopic hematuria, red cell casts, and proteinuria; the exception is membranous lupus nephritis, in which proteinuria is the dominant finding. Drug-induced lupus rarely leads to renal disease. Anti-dsDNA antibodies at high titer put the patient at risk for severe nephritis. Renal biopsy is not necessary in SLE patients whose renal function is rapidly deteriorating when they have an active sediment. If such patients fail to respond to the prompt initiation of glucocorticoid therapy demanded in such a situation, then biopsy should be undertaken. Patients with mild clinical disease should have a biopsy to determine if they have active, severe, inflammatory lesions, which might respond to therapy.

104. PROGNOSIS: INITIAL WORKUP: ANSWER: A

(Isselbacher, 13/e, pp 1667-1668.) This rare disorder is thought to be an autoimmune disease as 50 percent of patients will have antibodies to human oral mucous membrane. Ulcerations of the oral cavity, vagina, and external genitalia are common manifestations and usually resolve spontaneously in 1 to 2 weeks and heal without scarring. Involvement of the eye is serious, as rapid progression to blindness is a real possibility. Though 25 percent of patients develop peripheral vein thrombosis, pulmonary emboli are rare. The syndrome typically will resolve completely without long-term sequelae or early mortality.

105. HEALTH MAINTENANCE: CONTINUED CARE: ANSWER: A

(Carr, pp 420, 525.) Dysmenorrhea is considered secondary if associated with pelvic disease such as endometriosis, uterine myomas, or pelvic inflammatory disease. Primary dysmenorrhea is associated with a normal pelvic examination and with ovulatory cycles. The pain is usually accompanied by other symptoms—nausea, fatigue, diarrhea, and headache—which may be related to excess of prostaglandin $F_{2\alpha}$. The two major drug therapies effective in dysmenorrhea are oral contraceptives and antiprostaglandins. Treatment will reduce the number of women incapacitated by menstrual symptoms to about 10 percent of those treated. Contrary to past beliefs, psychologic factors play only a minor role in dysmenorrhea.

106. CLINICAL THERAPEUTICS: CONTINUED CARE: ANSWER: B

(Isselbacher, 13/e, chap 310. Pizzo, Am J Med 76:436, 1984.) If not attacked promptly, infection in neutropenic patients can be quickly fatal. Often, these patients display neither the signs nor the symptoms of infection. Fever should be regarded as an indication of infection, and antibiotic therapy should begin immediately after appropriate cultures are obtained. An effective initial antibiotic regimen would consist of a cephalosporin, carbenicillin, and gentamicin. Gammaglobulin is of little benefit in the treatment of cancer patients. Granulocyte transfusions and amphotericin administration may be of benefit in selected cases.

107. DIAGNOSIS: CONTINUED CARE: ANSWER: E

(Isselbacher, 13/e, chaps 286, 287. Kelly, chap 76, pp 1211-1230.) Systemic sclerosis can be classified into two variants depending on whether scleroderma is present only in the fingers (sclerodactyly) or whether it is also present proximal to the metacarpophalangeal joints. The former disorder is associated with a constellation of findings labeled the CREST syndrome: calcinosis, Raynaud's phenomenon, esophageal dysmotility, sclerodactyly, and telangiectasia. Although once thought not to be associated with significant internal organ involvement, the CREST variant of systemic sclerosis has occurred in association with involvement of the lungs, heart, and kidneys, in this respect resembling systemic sclerosis associated with proximal scleroderma. The fluorescent antinuclear antibody (ANA) test is positive in 40 to 80 percent of persons with systemic sclerosis. Antibodies are produced to deoxyribonucleoprotein, nucleolar, centromere, and topoisomerase 1 antigens.

Mixed connective-tissue disease is the overlap of three rheumatic disease syndromes: systemic lupus erythematosus (SLE), polymyositis, and the CREST variant of systemic sclerosis. It is associated with high titers of antinuclear antibodies directed against the extractable nuclear antigen ribonucleoprotein. Arthritis and a positive ANA are not sufficient to make a diagnosis of SLE. Overlap syndromes are diseases that fulfill diagnostic criteria for two rheumatic diseases. In the case described, symptoms and signs were insufficient to fulfill the diagnostic criteria for more than one rheumatic syndrome.

108. PROGNOSIS: CONTINUED CARE: ANSWER: A
(Isselbacher, 13/e, chap 59. Young, Clin Haematol 9:483, 1980.) Severe neutropenia is a rare idiosyncratic reaction to certain drugs, including propylthiouracil. In addition to having sore throat and oral and anal mucosal ulcerations, affected persons are susceptible to overwhelming, life-threatening infections. However, in the absence of fever or clinical signs of infection, they should be followed as outpatients, saving them exposure to nosocomial pathogens in the hospital. Empirical use of broad-spectrum antibiotics without fever or other signs of infection is not advisable, and corticosteroid therapy is not useful. White blood cell transfusion can be accompanied by serious morbidity (particularly, pulmonary leukostasis) and should be reserved for persons with transient neutropenia and documented septicemia. Because severe drug-induced neutropenia is generally self-limited once use of the offending drug has been stopped, consideration of bone marrow transplantation is not justified.

109. PROGNOSIS: INITIAL WORKUP: ANSWER: D
(Brooks, pp 263-279.) The vast majority of pancreatic carcinomas are located in the head of the gland. Patients may present with painless jaundice by virtue of the carcinoma's obstruction of the intrapancreatic portion of the common bile duct. It is in this group of patients that resection is even possible—although most will be unresectable. Tumors in the body or tail of the gland are universally unresectable. The cause of pancreatic cancer is not known. There is a very strong association with diabetes mellitus but the nature of this relationship is not known. Prognosis is uniformly dismal whether resection is done or not and only an anecdotal survivor will be alive at 5-year follow-up.

110. PROGNOSIS: CONTINUED CARE: ANSWER: E
(Eden, pp 693-719.) Maternal diabetes mellitus can affect a pregnant woman and her fetus in many ways. The development of preeclampsia or eclampsia is about four times as likely as among nondiabetic women. Infection also is more likely not only to occur but also to be severe. The incidences of fetal macrosomia or death and of dystocia are increased; and hydramnios is common. The likelihood of postpartum hemorrhage after vaginal delivery and the frequency of cesarean section both are increased in diabetic women.

111. APPLYING BASIC CONCEPTS: CONTINUED CARE: ANSWER: E
(Isselbacher, 13/e, chap 305. Lee, Semin Hematol 20:61, 1983.) A mild-to-moderate degree of anemia often accompanies chronic infectious, inflammatory, or neoplastic diseases. Typically, the anemia of chronic disease is normochromic and normocytic to microcytic. Bone marrow examination reveals normal erythroid maturation. Neither significant disturbance of hemoglobin synthesis nor hemolysis occurs in this type of anemia. Affected persons usually have a low serum iron concentration and a low total transferrin level (resulting in essentially normal or only slightly decreased fractional transferrin saturation). Even though storage iron is abundant, there is a decreased amount of iron in erythroblasts, reflecting a defect in the transfer of reticuloendothelial iron to developing red blood cells.

112. DIAGNOSTIC STUDIES: INITIAL WORKUP: ANSWER: D
(Isselbacher, 13/e, chap 315.) The presence of nonspecific anticoagulants (lupus-type) may predispose patients to thrombosis and is also associated with habitual abortions in some women. Patients with congenital dysfibrinogenemias may have variable results on screening coagulation tests. They often have slight prolongations in the prothrombin times or partial thromboplastin times, prolonged thrombin times, and a disparity between functional and immunologic assays of fibrinogen. Despite these abnormalities, patients may have either no symptoms or moderate bleeding, and a few dysfibrinogenemias have been associated with hypercoagulability. Congenital deficiencies of antithrombin III and protein C are familial thrombotic disorders and are not associated with abnormalities of the various clotting times. Factor XI deficiency is an autosomal recessive disorder often associated with bleeding following trauma or during the perioperative period.

113. HEALTH MAINTENANCE: CONTINUED CARE: ANSWER: C
(Isselbacher, 13/e, chap 307. Rosse, Clin Haematol 14:105, 1985.) Paroxysmal nocturnal hemoglobinuria, an acquired disorder of the bone marrow stem cell, affects not only red blood cells but also platelets and granulocytes. Like related myeloproliferative disorders (e.g., chronic myelogenous leukemia, essential thrombocythemia, polycythemia vera, myeloid metaplasia, and myelofibrosis), paroxysmal nocturnal hemoglobinuria may lead to acute myelogenous leukemia. Lymphoma, particularly involving the central nervous system, may develop in renal transplant recipients on immunosuppressive therapy as well as in persons with Wiskott-Aldrich syndrome. Persons who have Hodgkin's disease and have been treated with both radiation therapy and chemotherapy are at risk for developing leukemia. Acquired idiopathic refractory sideroblastic anemia leads to acute leukemia in about 10 percent of cases, but this phenomenon does not occur in hereditary forms of sideroblastic anemia.

114. DIAGNOSTIC STUDIES: INITIAL WORKUP: ANSWER: D
(Isselbacher, 13/e, chap 137. Steere, N Engl J Med 321:586, 1989.) In a patient with Lyme disease, biopsy of the typical skin lesion, erythema chronicum migrans, usually shows nondiagnostic perivascular lymphocytic and histiocytic infiltration. Though hematogenous dissemination of the spirochete that causes Lyme disease, *Borrelia burgdorferi*, does occur, it is rarely detected on direct examination. The spirochete has been cultured from blood, skin, and cerebrospinal fluid (CSF), but culture of this organism is not a routine procedure. Frank meningitis with CSF pleocytosis rarely occurs until several weeks or months into the illness. Lymphocytosis and an elevated protein level are typically found but are not diagnostic. The most useful study is a serum determination of IgG antibody titers, which are almost uniformly elevated after several weeks of illness.

115. CLINICAL INTERVENTION: CONTINUED CARE: ANSWER: D
(Isselbacher, 13/e, chap 108.) *Clostridium difficile* can be isolated on selective agar media, but this method is not dependable for diagnosis. Pseudomembranous colitis (PMC) is caused by the local action of at least two enterotoxins, toxins A and B. Serologic tests are not helpful. The punctate plaques on a hyperemic mucosa are characteristic of PMC, but similar pathologic changes can be seen with ischemic colitis. The best diagnostic test is the demonstration of *C. difficile* cytotoxin, an assay that can be positive in 24 h. Clostridia are part of normal fecal flora, so a Gram stain of the stool would not be helpful.

116. CLINICAL INTERVENTION: CONTINUED CARE: ANSWER: E
(Isselbacher, 13/e, p 1426.) These tumors are usually large at diagnosis and often sessile. They are 3 times more likely to harbor malignancy than other tubular adenomas. They are most often located in the distal colon but can be encountered in the cecum or proximal gut. The adenoma is the histologic type of colon polyp found in the familial polyposis syndrome.

117. APPLYING BASIC CONCEPTS: INITIAL WORKUP: ANSWERS: A, C, E
(Isselbacher, 13/e, p 2394.) Lambert-Eaton syndrome is associated with decreased reflexes. It can be associated with an underlying malignant tumor or the subsequent development of one, but is not a predisposing factor in the development of neoplasia.

118. CLINICAL INTERVENTION: CONTINUED CARE: ANSWERS: A, D
(Isselbacher, 13/e, pp 1375-1377.) Zollinger-Ellison syndrome is due to excessive gastric acid production that occurs in response to the abnormally high levels of gastrin secreted from gastrinomas. These islet cell tumors are usually pancreatic in origin (though duodenal gastrinomas likely account for many previously undetected gastrinomas), multiple (50 to 67 percent), and malignant (90 percent). Half of patients with MEN I will have gastrinomas as well as hyperplasia, adenomas, or carcinomas of the parathyroid and pituitary glands. The hypersecretion of gastrin acts on the parietal cells in the stomach to produce excess gastric acid. This results in peptic ulceration of the stomach and duodenum in a distribution that is usually similar to non-Zollinger-Ellison-related peptic ulcer disease. Multiple ulcers occur in 25 percent of patients and involve the postbulbar duodenum and jejunum. Complete surgical resection of the gastrinoma(s) is the optimal treatment. If this is not achievable, treatment with omperazole is used to block gastric acid production.

119. APPLYING BASIC CONCEPTS: INITIAL WORKUP: ANSWER: E
(Isselbacher, 13/e, chap 385.) Oculopharyngeal dystrophy is a dominantly inherited disease occurring in families of French-Canadian or middle-European ancestry. Because it causes late-onset progressive ptosis and difficulty with swallowing, it may be difficult to distinguish from myasthenia gravis, which is not a dystrophic muscle disease. Proximal weakness and ophthalmoplegia suggest the presence of a progressive external ophthalmoplegia.

120. APPLYING BASIC CONCEPTS: INITIAL WORKUP: ANSWERS: A, C, D
(Isselbacher, 13/e, pp 2385-2387.) Oculopharyngeal dystrophy is characterized by ophthalmoplegia, pharyngeal weakness that can lead to dysphagia and aspiration, and neck weakness. The disorder is transmitted genetically with autosomal dominant inheritance and complete penetration. Foot-drop is a feature of facioscapulohumeral muscular dystrophy, not oculopharyngeal dystrophy.

121. CLINICAL THERAPEUTICS: EMERGENCY: ANSWER: C
(Isselbacher, 13/e, chap 113.) Legionnaire's disease is caused by *Legionella pneumophila*. Person-to-person spread of this soil organism has not been documented. Gastrointestinal symptoms preceding pneumonia are sometimes a clue to the diagnosis. In many cases, chest x-ray shows dense infiltrates despite a paucity of physical signs, such as rales or rhonchi; in this regard, the disease resembles *Mycoplasma* pneumonia. Although *L. pneumophila* has been found in vitro to be sensitive to several drugs, erythromycin is the treatment of choice.

122. CLINICAL THERAPEUTICS: EMERGENCY: ANSWER: D
(Isselbacher, 13/e, chap 152.) The man described in the question has symptoms suggesting influenza complicated by bacterial pneumonia. Pneumococci and staphylococci are the leading pathogens causing secondary bacterial infection in this situation, and effective therapy would include drugs that act against penicillinase-producing staphylococci. The agent of choice is nafcillin or another semisynthetic penicillinase-resistant penicillin; penicillin G would be an ill-advised choice. Other drugs acceptable as alternative therapies would include vancomycin, clindamycin, and cephalothin.

123. CLINICAL THERAPEUTICS: CONTINUED CARE: ANSWER: C
(Isselbacher, 13/e, chap 142.) Acyclovir is now the drug of choice in the treatment of herpes encephalitis. It has been shown to be more effective than vidarabine and also has fewer side effects. Acyclovir has been shown both to shorten viral shedding in mucocutaneous infections and to prevent outbreaks in immunocompromised patients. Similarly, acyclovir is useful in immunocompromised patients with herpes zoster, but it is not yet indicated in nonimmunocompromised patients in whom the risk of dissemination is very small. Both the frequency and the duration of recurrent episodes of genital herpes are reduced on long-term suppressive therapy. As soon as the drug is discontinued, however, infection recurs.

124. CLINICAL THERAPEUTICS: CONTINUED CARE: ANSWER: A
(Schwartz, 6/e, p 71.) Reduction of an elevated serum potassium level is important to avoid the cardiovascular complications that ultimately culminate in diastolic cardiac arrest. Kayexalate is a cation exchange resin that is instilled into the gastrointestinal tract and exchanges sodium for potassium ions. Its use is limited to semiacute and chronic potassium elevations. Sodium bicarbonate causes a rise in serum pH and shifts potassium intracellularly. Administration of glucose initiates glycogen synthesis and uptake of potassium. Insulin can be used in conjunction with this to aid in the shift of potassium intracellularly. Calcium gluconate does not affect the serum potassium level but rather counteracts the myocardial effects of hyperkalemia.

125. DIAGNOSIS: EMERGENCY: ANSWER: C
(Isselbacher, 13/e, chap 206.) Acute pericarditis is associated with ST-segment elevation and, frequently, PR-segment depression. Usually, reciprocal ST-segment depression is not present. T waves begin to invert only after the ST segment becomes isoelectric. Elevations in serum creatine phosphokinase levels to twice normal may be associated with uncomplicated pericarditis.

126. DIAGNOSTIC STUDIES: CONTINUED CARE: ANSWER: D
(Carr, pp 439-440, 508-509.) A hysterosalpingogram is a procedure in which 3 to 6 mL of either an oil- or water-soluble contrast medium is injected through the cervix in order to outline the uterine cavity and fallopian tubes. Spill of contrast medium into the peritoneal cavity proves patency of the uterine cavity and fallopian tubes. By outlining the cavity, abnormalities such as bicornuate uterus, uterine polyps, submucous myomas, salpingitis isthmica nodosum, and hydrosalpinx can be identified. Some controlled studies have shown a therapeutic effect resulting in an increased rate of pregnancy in infertility patients.

127. DIAGNOSTIC STUDIES: CONTINUED CARE: ANSWER: A

(Kase, 2/e, pp 465-469.) A positive pregnancy test would confirm the presence of a pregnancy. The culdocentesis is useful in finding non-clotting blood when there is intraperitoneal bleeding from an ectopic pregnancy. Ultrasound can rule out an ectopic pregnancy by finding an intrauterine pregnancy. A pelvic examination could detect an adnexal mass. The findings on an abdominal flat plate would be nonspecific in an ectopic pregnancy.

128. LEGAL AND ETHICAL ISSUES: CONTINUED CARE: ANSWER: D

(Eden, pp 921-931.) Negligence law governs conduct and embraces acts of both commission and omission, i.e., what a person did or failed to do. In general the law expects all persons to conduct themselves in a fashion that does not expose others to an unreasonable risk of harm. In a fiduciary relationship such as physician-patient, the physician is held to a higher standard of behavior because of the imbalance of knowledge. In general, the real gist of negligence is not carelessness or ineptitude, but rather how unreasonable the risk of harm the patient was exposed to by the physician's action. Thus physicians are held accountable to a standard of care that asks the question, "What would the reasonable physician do under this specific set of circumstances?" One is not held accountable to the level of the leading experts in any given field, but rather the prevailing standards among average practitioners. When a doctor-patient relationship is established, the defendant owes a duty to the patient. If the defendant breaches that duty, i.e., acts in a way that is inconsistent with the standard of care and that can be shown to have caused damage directly to the patient (proximate damage), then the physician may be held liable for compensation.

129. CLINICAL INTERVENTION: CONTINUED CARE: ANSWER: B

(Ryan, 5/e, pp 50, 718-719.) Ovulation is not affected in Asherman syndrome. Because of the decreased amount of functional endometrium, hypomenorrhea or amenorrhea is common. The best diagnostic study is the hysterosalpingogram under fluoroscopy. Hysteroscopy with lysis of adhesions is the treatment of choice. Prophylactic antibiotics may improve success rates.

130. CLINICAL THERAPEUTICS: CONTINUED CARE: ANSWER: A

(Isselbacher, 13/e, chap 82.) Since BCG is a live attenuated organism and has been reported to cause disseminated infection in immunocompromised patients, it should not be administered to those with HIV infection or others with suspected immunodeficiency. Though patients with immune dysfunction often do not mount a good response to an administered vaccine, they should still receive certain preparations. Patients about to undergo splenectomy or cancer chemotherapy should, when possible, be vaccinated prior to therapy. Influenza vaccine should be given in autumn to those with any chronic medical illness in addition to those with obvious immune deficiency. The chronically ill, the immunosuppressed, and those at risk for infection with encapsulated microorganisms (anatomic or functional asplenia, multiple myeloma) should receive pneumococcal vaccine. The last group plus those with terminal complement component deficiencies should receive the quadrivalent meningococcal vaccine. Patients with HIV infection, especially those who are potential household contacts of children who are receiving the oral polio vaccine (attenuated live virus), should receive three doses of the inactivated polio vaccine.

131. CLINICAL INTERVENTION: CONTINUED CARE: ANSWER: D

(Eden, pp 749-765.) Prior to the use of Rh_0 immunoglobulin in the nonsensitized Rh-negative woman who delivered an Rh-positive infant, the isoimmunization rate was about 10 percent. Its use is also recommended in Rh-negative, nonsensitized women after abortion, molar pregnancy, ectopic pregnancy, amniocentesis, and vaginal bleeding in pregnancy. Nearly 1.8 percent of Rh-negative women become sensitized during the third trimester. Administration of Rh_0 immunoglobulin at 28 to 32 weeks in the Rh-negative, nonsensitized woman has decreased the rate of sensitization to 0.07 percent.

132. CLINICAL INTERVENTION: CONTINUED CARE: ANSWER: E

(Isselbacher, 13/e, chap 203.) PTCA is now widely used to revascularize suitable coronary lesions. Although adequate dilation is achieved in more than 85 percent of patients, recurrent stenosis develops in approximately 20 percent within 6 months. Angioplasty has been successfully performed on obstructive lesions within bypass grafts and in patients with recent total occlusion (within 3 months) of native coronaries. Significant left main artery disease ordinarily remains a contraindication to the procedure, coronary artery bypass grafting appears to be safer at present. The success rate of repeated PTCA is actually better than that of the first procedure.

133. HISTORY AND PHYSICAL: INITIAL WORKUP: ANSWER: C

(Isselbacher, 13/e, chap 296.) Osteoarthritis, the most common joint disease, is diagnosed on the basis of clinical and laboratory features. One of the earliest x-ray findings is joint space narrowing as periarticular cartilage is lost. A joint involved with osteoarthritis may be tender or slightly swollen; significant effusions are rare. The sensation of bone rubbing against bone (bony crepitus) may be elicited upon movement of an affected joint. Bony prominences on both the distal interphalangeal joints (Heberden's nodes) and the proximal interphalangeal joints (Bouchard's nodes) are commonly seen. Osteoarthritis in the patellofemoral joint may manifest as a positive "shrug" sign, i.e., pain when the patella is manually compressed against the femur when the quadriceps contract. In contrast, rheumatoid arthritis (RA) commonly involves the proximal interphalangeal joint. Moreover, destruction of ligaments and tendons seen in RA may result in characteristic hand changes such as hyperextension of the proximal interphalangeal joints with compensatory flexion of the distal interphalangeal joints (swan-neck deformity) or flexion deformity of the proximal interphalangeals and extension of the distal interphalangeals (boutonnière deformity).

134. APPLYING BASIC CONCEPTS: INITIAL WORKUP: ANSWER: B

(Isselbacher, 13/e, pp 1728-1730.) Megaloblastic anemia can be considered to be due to a deficiency of cobalamin or folic acid. Intrinsic factor, produced in the stomach, is necessary for the absorption of cobalamin. Gastrectomy or diffuse gastric injury following corrosive ingestion can result in inadequate cobalamin and megaloblastic anemia. Acidification of the small bowel contents, as occurs in the Zollinger-Ellison syndrome, may cause malabsorption of cobalamin. Tropical sprue is associated with megaloblastic anemia because of interference of distal ileal resorption of cobalamin or folic acid malabsorption. It is an unusual complication of non-tropical sprue. Poor folic acid intake, as in alcoholism, or increased folic acid consumption, as in pregnancy, can result in megaloblastic anemia. Folate supplements are important in pregnancy as fetal neural tube defects are associated with folic acid deficiency.

135. APPLYING BASIC CONCEPTS: INITIAL WORKUP: ANSWER: E

(Isselbacher, 13/e, chap 102.) The pathogenicity of staphylococci is related to a number of biologic properties, including the production of coagulase, catalase, exotoxin, and enterotoxin. Coagulase and catalase are thought to protect staphylococci within a host from being destroyed by phagocytes. Some staphylococcal strains produce exotoxins that can cause intraepidermal cleavage and bullae formation, as well as toxic shock syndrome. Other strains elaborate an enterotoxin that produces gastrointestinal disease. The production of penicillinase, though rendering a pathogenic organism harder to destroy pharmacologically, does not contribute to pathogenicity.

136. HEALTH MAINTENANCE: CONTINUED CARE: ANSWER: B

(Eden, pp 269-279. Evans, pp 225-229.) All the listed factors are important in MSAFP screening. However, maternal age is not used as a criterion in determining the multiple of the median (MOM), but is used once the MOM has been determined. The maternal age determines what the cutoff point is for calling a value abnormal. Because AFP is a fetal product, if it is distributed over a larger mother, the effective serum concentration is lower. Therefore a maternal weight correction is used to adjust for differing plasma volumes. The race of the patient is important because, for reasons that are unclear, black patients have a slightly higher level of MSAFP than do white patients despite the fact that the risk of neural tube defects in the black population is lower than that of white patients. A separate database for black and white patients is the most optimal way of handling such data. Gestational age is important because AFP values normally rise in maternal serum with advancing gestational age. A significant discrepancy between a patient's opinion of gestational age and actual gestational age may explain a seemingly abnormal result. Multiple gestations are important because if there are two or more fetuses, the value of AFP seen normally will be higher. In most programs an upper cutoff point of 4.5 MOM is used for known twins, and a lower cutoff point of 1.0 MOM is common for increased risk of chromosomal abnormalities.

137. HEALTH MAINTENANCE: INITIAL WORKUP: ANSWER: D

(Davis, pp 2348-2349.) Signs and symptoms of the carpal tunnel syndrome are related to the distribution of the median nerve. This nerve, which passes through the carpal tunnel in the wrist with the finger flexor tendons, may suffer compression from fibrous scarring or malalignment following a fracture of the wrist. Nerve compression may also occur in patients with rheumatoid arthritis who develop flexor tenosynovitis. In women, the syndrome frequently first appears during pregnancy and recurs during the premenstrual phase of subsequent menstrual cycles. In these cases, symptoms are presumably the result of the effects of fluid retention and pressure on the median nerve owing to tissue swelling. In many instances, symptoms are limited to nocturnal pain and paresthesias.

138. APPLYING BASIC CONCEPTS: INITIAL WORKUP: ANSWER: D
139. APPLYING BASIC CONCEPTS: INITIAL WORKUP: ANSWER: A

(Isselbacher, 13/e, p 1338.) Wilms tumor has been classically divided into favorable and unfavorable histologic groups which have therapeutic and prognostic implications. The vast majority of the tumors have favorable histology. Angiomyolipomas are frequently associated with tuberous sclerosis and can be multiple and diffusely infiltrate both kidneys with small fat-containing tumors.

140. CLINICAL THERAPEUTICS: INITIAL WORKUP: ANSWER: B
141. CLINICAL THERAPEUTICS: INITIAL WORKUP: ANSWER: A
(Isselbacher, 13/e, TABLE 245-1, p 1330.)

142. CLINICAL THERAPEUTICS: CONTINUED CARE: ANSWER: D
143. CLINICAL THERAPEUTICS: CONTINUED CARE: ANSWER: E
(Hardy, 2/e, pp 250-255.) Morphine is a potent narcotic agent. Its use during general anesthesia can potentiate the analgesic effects of the inhalation agents. It causes histamine release with the risk of hypotension if given in a large bolus dose.
Nitrous oxide (N_2O) is a frequently used inhalation analgesic. However, because the MAC (minimum alveolar anesthetic concentration) is so high (over 100), true anesthesia at one atmosphere pressure cannot be obtained without compromising oxygen delivery to the patient. Since nitrous oxide is thirty times more soluble than nitrogen in blood, it enters a collection of trapped air at a rate faster than nitrogen leaves the collection. Thus, the trapped air will increase in volume. If the trapped air is a result of bowel obstruction, intestinal distention will increase.

144. CLINICAL THERAPEUTICS: CONTINUED CARE: ANSWER: D
145. CLINICAL THERAPEUTICS: CONTINUED CARE: ANSWER: D
146. CLINICAL THERAPEUTICS: CONTINUED CARE: ANSWER: E
(Isselbacher, 13/e, chap 367.) Rash and idiosyncratic bone marrow suppression are at times seen with phenytoin. Hepatotoxicity is a rare but feared effect of carbamazepine and an acute effect of valproic acid. In addition to the side effects listed in the question, phenytoin causes the appearance of a slightly prognathic jaw and coarsened facies. Phenytoin's neurologic side effects include ataxia. In fact, ataxia is a potential side effect of virtually all the anticonvulsants, including each of those listed in the question.

147. DIAGNOSIS: EMERGENCY: ANSWER: B
148. HISTORY AND PHYSICAL: EMERGENCY: ANSWER: C
(Schwartz, 6/e, pp 1900-1934.) Dislocation of the radial head with a fracture of the proximal third of the ulna is known as Monteggia's deformity. Usually, the radial head is dislocated anteriorly. The injury is usually caused by forced pronation. The injury can be treated by reduction and stabilization of the ulna followed by reduction of the radial head via supination and direct pressure. A spiral fracture, frequently seen in the tibia in skiers, results from the application of torque to a long bone. Greenstick fractures are common in children. The bones of young children are able to bend to a greater degree than those of adults; the fracture may occur only at the site of maximal cortical stress but not at the opposite cortex, the site of maximal longitudinal compression. Fractures of the navicular bone of the wrist should be suspected in anyone, particularly a young person, who falls on an outstretched hand. Although x-rays are mandatory, it is important to realize that the fracture may not be seen on the initial x-ray and that a presumptive diagnosis can and should be made on clinical grounds alone. Typically, there will be tenderness to palpation over the navicular tuberosity and limitation of wrist flexion and extension. Immobilization of the wrist for about 16 weeks and sometimes up to 6 months is required.

149. CLINICAL THERAPEUTICS: CONTINUED CARE: ANSWER: E
150. CLINICAL THERAPEUTICS: CONTINUED CARE: ANSWER: B
(Isselbacher, 13/e, chap 318.) Vinblastine and vincristine are plant alkaloids. They cause metaphase arrest in dividing cells by binding directly to tubulin; in addition, they interfere with the assembly of spindle proteins.
5-Fluorouracil, a pyrimidine analogue, blocks thymidylate synthetase, an enzyme important in the synthesis of thymidylate and DNA. Its active form is the metabolite 5-fluorodeoxyuridine monophosphate.

151. HISTORY AND PHYSICAL: CONTINUED CARE: ANSWER: C
152. HISTORY AND PHYSICAL: EMERGENCY: ANSWER: D
153. HISTORY AND PHYSICAL: EMERGENCY: ANSWER: D
(Isselbacher, 13/e, chap 192.) Slow *y* descent is due to delayed atrial emptying. This phenomenon occurs in mitral or tricuspid stenosis, atrial myxomas, and cor triatriatum. Acute mitral regurgitation is associated with tall regurgitant *v* waves, which reflect regurgitation of blood into a noncompliant left atrium during systole. They are often absent in more chronic mitral regurgitation—a dilated left atrium can accommodate large volumes of blood without a significant increase in pressure. A regurgitant *v* wave often slightly precedes the usual physiologic *v* wave, which reflects venous return to the atria while atrioventricular valves are closed. In ventricular septal rupture with left-to-right shunt, venous return to the left atrium increases and the *v* wave becomes exaggerated.

154. DIAGNOSTIC STUDIES: CONTINUED CARE: ANSWER: D
155. HISTORY AND PHYSICAL: INITIAL WORKUP: ANSWER: A
(Isselbacher, 13/e, pp 1361-1362.) The nodular plaques seen in *Candida* esophagitis are due to the yeast itself and adjacent inflammation. *Herpes simplex* virus induces superficial erosions and associated vesicular lesions in the esophagus. Both *Herpes simplex* virus and *Candida* esophagitis typically occur in immunocompromised patients. Radiation esophagitis can occur following mediastinal radiation and can be potentiated by chemotherapeutic agents including bleomycin, doxorubicin and cyclophosphamide. Doxycycline, tetracycline and clindamycin are frequent causes of pill-induced esophagitis. KCl, aspirin, and ferrous sulphate are also common medications which are associated with this form of erosive esophagitis.

156. HISTORY AND PHYSICAL: INITIAL WORKUP: ANSWER: D
157. HISTORY AND PHYSICAL: INITIAL WORKUP: ANSWER: B
(Isselbacher, 13/e, TABLE 274-6, p 1531.)

158. APPLYING BASIC CONCEPTS: CONTINUED CARE: ANSWER: A
159. APPLYING BASIC CONCEPTS: CONTINUED CARE: ANSWER: D
(Isselbacher, 13/e, chap 81.) Several distinct infectious syndromes have been linked to specific deficits in host defenses. Patients with AIDS are susceptible to multiple infections against which intact cellular immunity is required. *Pneumocystis carinii* is the most frequent infection, but cytomegalovirus, *Mycobacterium avium-intracellulare*, and cryptococcal infections are also common. In Chédiak-Higashi syndrome, a defect in neutrophil chemotaxis and phagocytosis results in recurrent staphylococcal infections.

160. DIAGNOSIS: CONTINUED CARE: ANSWER: A

161. DIAGNOSIS: CONTINUED CARE: ANSWER: D

(Eden, pp 749-766. Evans, pp 44-55, 60-71.) Rh sensitization that causes severe fetal anemia could lead to hydrops fetalis, a severe subcutaneous edema and effusion into serous cavities, such as into the abdominal cavity, that causes ascites. Portal hypertension, severe hypoalbuminemia, and heart failure contribute to the ascites. Assuming that the dates are correct, the most common reason for an elevated level of maternal serum alpha-fetoprotein is an open defect of the neural tube such as open spina bifida or anencephaly. At the same time that an ultrasound examination is obtained, an amniocentesis is also done to look for elevated levels in amniotic fluid.

162. HISTORY AND PHYSICAL: CONTINUED CARE: ANSWER: E

163. HISTORY AND PHYSICAL: CONTINUED CARE: ANSWER: B

(Isselbacher, 13/e, chaps 199, 222.) Many hereditary conditions and exposures to infectious agents during pregnancy result in congenital heart disease. Maternal rubella during pregnancy can result in deafness, microcephaly, and cataracts in the infant. The most common cardiovascular lesions are pulmonic stenosis, multiple pulmonary artery stenoses, and patent ductus arteriosus. Cystic fibrosis is an autosomal recessive disease primarily affecting exocrine glands and results in chronic obstructive lung disease and pancreatic insufficiency. The prominent abnormalities of lung function may result in cor pulmonale.

164. DIAGNOSTIC STUDIES: CONTINUED CARE: ANSWER: A

165. DIAGNOSTIC STUDIES: CONTINUED CARE: ANSWER: D

(Isselbacher, 13/e, TABLE 307-2, p 1746.)

166. CLINICAL INTERVENTION: CONTINUED CARE: ANSWER: D

167. CLINICAL INTERVENTION: CONTINUED CARE: ANSWER: B

(Isselbacher, 13/e, pp 325, 1621, 1773, 1777.) Cytoplasmic extensions noted occasionally on smear and consistently with phase microscopy give a "hairy" appearance to cells. The Reed-Sternberg cell rarely can be seen in non-Hodgkin lymphomas but is the hallmark of Hodgkin's disease. The lytic defects and osteoporosis seen with myeloma are due to the osteoclast activating factor produced by the myeloma cells. Diseases associated with a proliferation of either tissue macrophages (histiocytes) or special bone marrow-derived cells called Langerhans' cells are termed hystiocytoses.

168. DIAGNOSTIC STUDIES: CONTINUED CARE: ANSWER: C

169. DIAGNOSTIC STUDIES: CONTINUED CARE: ANSWER: B

(Isselbacher, 13/e, chaps 201, 204, 206.) Right heart failure, or elevated right-heart filling pressure, can develop from many causes. Right heart failure most commonly occurs as a result of pulmonary artery hypertension. Pulmonary artery hypertension, in turn, arises either from increased pulmonary vascular resistance with lung disease, in which case the pulmonary capillary wedge pressure (left atrial pressure) is not elevated, or from left-sided failure or valvular disease, in which case left atrial pressure is increased. Massive right ventricular infarction can cause the right side of the heart to fail at low systolic pressures. With primary myocardial disease, both left and right atrial pressures are elevated; however, when diastolic pressures are equal in the left and right cardiac chambers, external compression, such as constrictive pericarditis, must be suspected as the cause.

170. DIAGNOSTIC STUDIES: INITIAL WORKUP: ANSWER: C

171. DIAGNOSTIC STUDIES: INITIAL WORKUP: ANSWER: A

(Schwartz, 6/e, pp 103-108.) Prothrombin time measures the speed of coagulation in the extrinsic pathway. A tissue source of procoagulant (thromboplastin) with calcium is added to plasma. The test will detect deficiencies in factors II, V, VII, X, and fibrinogen and is used to monitor patients receiving coumarin derivatives. However, even small amounts of heparin will artificially prolong the clotting time so that accurate prothrombin times can only be obtained when the patient has not received heparin for at least 5 h.

The intrinsic pathway is measured by the partial thromboplastin time. This test is sensitive for defects in factors VIII, IX, XI, XII, and all the factors of the extrinsic pathway and is used to monitor the status of patients on heparin.

The bleeding time assesses the interaction of platelets and the formation of the platelet plug. Therefore it will pick up deficiencies in both qualitative and quantitative platelet function. Ingestion of aspirin within 1 week of the test will alter the result.

The thrombin time assesses qualitative abnormalities in fibrinogen and the presence of inhibitors to fibrin polymerization. A standard amount of fibrin is added to a fixed volume of plasma and clotting time is measured.

172. HEALTH MAINTENANCE: INITIAL WORKUP: ANSWER: D

173. HEALTH MAINTENANCE: INITIAL WORKUP: ANSWER: C

(Isselbacher, 13/e, pp 1819, 2339.) Certain hereditary conditions predispose to the development of neoplasia. The neurocutaneous disorders (Choices A, B, and C) are well known for this. Neurofibromatosis is highly associated with benign and malignant neural tumors, as well as glial tumors and meningiomas. Von Hippel-Lindau disease is associated with cerebellar hemangioblastomas, retinal angiomas, and renal cell carcinoma. Both disorders also have an association with pheochromocytomas. Tuberous sclerosis is characterized by glial tumors as well as renal angiomyofibromas and cardiac rhabdomyomas. Ataxia-telangiectasia is associated with lymphomas and leukemias. The increased incidence of malignancy in this disorder is felt to be due to chromosomal fragility.

174. APPLYING BASIC CONCEPTS: INITIAL WORKUP: ANSWER: B
175. DIAGNOSIS: EMERGENCY: ANSWER: E
176. DIAGNOSIS: INITIAL WORKUP: ANSWER: A

(Schwartz, 6/e, pp 1881-1883, 1954-1956.) Osteosarcomas arise from osteoblasts and usually cause death within 2 years of diagnosis. They generally arise in long bones—particularly the femur—and initially cause pain. Later, local swelling and tenderness may appear. Overlying bone is irregularly eroded; the tumor may break the cortex and expand into adjacent soft tissue. Osteosarcomas may arise in bones affected by Paget's disease. Osteoid osteoma also arises from osteoblasts but is usually seen in males in their teens or twenties. Night pain, which responds only to aspirin, is the classic presenting symptom. Treatment is resection of the lesion, which is usually in the lower extremity or the spine. Osteochondromas, which are benign projections of bone covered by a cartilaginous cap, usually develop at the end of a long bone, most frequently from the tibia or femur near the knee. Arising during the second decade of life, they cease growing upon closure of the epiphyses and are asymptomatic unless they are subjected to trauma or impinge on sensitive tissue. Osteochondromas occasionally undergo malignant transformation. Unicameral bone cysts are single-chambered, benign lesions that most frequently occur as solitary lesions in the proximal humerus or femur. They frequently are associated with pathological fractures because of thinning of adjacent bone cortices. The cysts do not undergo malignant transformation. Treatment consists of scraping the cyst walls and packing with bone chips or removal of the entire segment of bone that contains a cyst (subperiosteal resection). Aneurysmal bone cysts, thought to arise from vascular tissue in bone, frequently cause local pain. Pathological fractures are commonly associated with these cysts and may be accompanied by heavy bleeding. Preferred surgical treatment consists of curettage and packing with bone chips. Radiation may induce vascular sclerosis in surgically inaccessible cysts.

177. DIAGNOSIS: EMERGENCY: ANSWER: E
178. DIAGNOSIS: EMERGENCY: ANSWER: A

(Evans, pp 136-140. Herbst, 2/e, pp 162, 449-453.) Bleeding occurs in about 30 to 40 percent of human gestations before 20 weeks of pregnancy with about half of these pregnancies ending in spontaneous abortion. A threatened abortion takes place when this uterine bleeding occurs without any cervical dilation or effacement.

In a patient bleeding during the first half of pregnancy, the diagnosis of inevitable abortion is strengthened if the bleeding is profuse and associated with uterine cramping pains. If cervical dilation has occurred, with or without rupture of membranes, the abortion is inevitable.

If only a portion of the products of conception has been expelled and the cervix remains dilated, a diagnosis of incomplete abortion is made. However, if all fetal and placental tissue has been expelled, the cervix is closed, bleeding from the canal is minimal or decreasing, and uterine cramps have ceased, a diagnosis of complete abortion can be made.

The diagnosis of missed abortion is suspected when the uterus fails to continue to enlarge with or without uterine bleeding or spotting. A missed abortion is one in which fetal death occurs before 20 weeks' gestation without expulsion of any fetal or maternal tissue for at least 8 weeks thereafter. When a fetus is retained in the uterus beyond 5 weeks after fetal death, consumptive coagulability with hypofibrogenemia may occur. This is uncommon, however, in gestations of less than 14 weeks' duration.

179. HEALTH MAINTENANCE: CONTINUED CARE: ANSWER: E
180. HEALTH MAINTENANCE: CONTINUED CARE: ANSWER: A

(Evans, pp 111-116.) Viral infections during pregnancy are of great concern. The risk to the fetus is greatest during the first trimester. Congenital infection in most instances results from transplacental transmission of the virus during maternal viremia. In addition, perinatal infection may result from acquisition of virus by passage of the infant through a contaminated birth canal. Cytomegalovirus, rubella, and varicella are well established as teratogens. Congenital disease may range from mild symptoms to major congenital defects to asymptomatic disease with late sequelae. Hepatitis B is only rarely transmitted in utero, but usually at the time of birth, and may cause a mild to severe hepatitis in infancy or, more commonly, result in a carrier state. Carriers run the risk of developing cirrhosis or hepatocellular carcinoma later in life. Rubeola is uncommon in pregnancy and has not been associated with any specific anomalies.

181. APPLYING BASIC CONCEPTS: INITIAL WORKUP: ANSWER: C
182. APPLYING BASIC CONCEPTS: INITIAL WORKUP: ANSWER: B

(Isselbacher, 13/e, TABLE 257-2, p 1425.)

183. HISTORY AND PHYSICAL: INITIAL WORKUP: ANSWER: E
184. CLINICAL THERAPEUTICS: CONTINUED CARE: ANSWER: A

(Ryan, 5/e, pp 117-121, 591-595.) Trichomonas vaginalis classically gives rise to a yellowish, frothy discharge, which is foul-smelling and causes pruritus. The pathognomonic "strawberry spots," which consist of punctate hemorrhagic spots on the vaginal mucosa, can sometimes be seen. The diagnosis is made by observing the characteristic motile protozoan on wet mounts. The mainstay of treatment is oral metronidazole, either in a single dose of 2 g or 250 mg three times a day for 7 to 10 days. Metronidazole has a disulfiram-like effect, and women taking it should refrain from consumption of alcohol. Vaginal suppositories of clotrimazole, 100 mg once a day for 7 days, are also effective and are preferred by some because of carcinogenicity associated with rodents treated with metronidazole.

Postmenopausal women who present with symptoms like itching, irritation secondary to dryness, and dyspareunia often have atrophic (senile) vaginitis. Owing to the lack of estrogen, the vaginal mucosa becomes very thin and easily irritable. This condition responds well to either oral intake of estrogen or local application of estrogen creams.

185. CLINICAL INTERVENTION: CONTINUED CARE: ANSWER: A
186. CLINICAL INTERVENTION: CONTINUED CARE: ANSWER: E

(Schwartz, 6/e, p 65.) One of the most common causes of dehydration and metabolic disarray in surgical patients is the failure to replace gastrointestinal losses. External losses can often be collected for measurement of volume and ionic composition. Accurate replacement of these measured losses is clearly the best method of avoiding imbalance. However, a knowledge of the ionic composition of the intestinal contents at various sites permits an accurate estimate for early replacement. Most of these secretions start as extracellular fluid (with a composition similar to that of plasma) and are modified by intestinal glands. The glands of the small intestine secrete various amounts of bicarbonate; the chloride content is depressed to an equivalent degree (to maintain ionic balance). Colonic contents (stool) and saliva are most notable for their potassium content. Stool also has a high bicarbonate content. Severe diarrhea can therefore cause potassium depletion and a metabolic acidosis.

187. DIAGNOSTIC STUDIES: CONTINUED CARE: ANSWER: D
188. DIAGNOSTIC STUDIES: INITIAL WORKUP: ANSWER: C

(Isselbacher, 13/e, pp 1495-1496.) Cavernous hemangioma is a common benign lesion of the liver characterized by endothelial-lined vascular spaces. These spaces will accumulate labeled RBCs and can be diagnosed definitively with nuclear imaging. Frequently, however, the diagnosis is suspected based on ultrasound or CT findings and no further diagnostic workup is needed. FNH is a benign liver mass that is unique among solid tumors of the liver in that it contains functioning Kupffer cells that will accumulate sulfur colloid. Thus, this lesion commonly will be "hot" or "warm" on sulfur colloid nuclear studies. Bile peritonitis may result from bile duct injury or inadequate cystic duct ligation that results in a communication between the biliary tree and the peritoneal space. The iminoacetic acid agents, the IDA family, will be taken up by the liver and excreted in the bile. These agents are useful in the detection of bile leaks. Because of the lipid solubility of xenon gas, there is increased deposition of this agent in the fatty liver. This is normally detected as an incidental finding on ventilation scintigrams, as xenon gas is the agent often used in pulmonary ventilation studies.

189. HEALTH MAINTENANCE: CONTINUED CARE: ANSWER: D
190. HEALTH MAINTENANCE: CONTINUED CARE: ANSWER: A

(Silverman, 8/e, pp 1072, 1279.) Kawasaki disease, or mucocutaneous lymph node syndrome, is an acute illness characterized by fever, desquamative rash of the palms and soles, conjunctivitis, and fissures around the mouth. The cervical lymph nodes are usually enlarged. Occasionally, patients develop coronary artery aneurysms as a delayed complication, which may cause coronary thrombosis or cardiac ischemia. Lymphocytic interstitial pneumonitis is a complication of AIDS that is more common in children than adults. The chest x-ray generally reveals a reticular-nodular pattern, but may have a more patchy (even lobar) distribution. With the reticular-nodular pattern, the differential diagnosis includes tuberculosis; however, these patients are usually not acutely ill.

Histiocytosis X refers to a spectrum of clinical diseases, including Letterer-Siwe, Hand-Schüller-Christian disease, and eosinophilic granuloma, which are caused by an abnormal proliferation of histiocytes. All three varieties of disease may involve the lung. Alveolar-wall invasion by histiocytes may result in pulmonary fibrosis and the development of multiple cysts. This may lead to end-stage "honeycomb lung."

191. DIAGNOSTIC STUDIES: INITIAL WORKUP: ANSWER: E
192. DIAGNOSTIC STUDIES: INITIAL WORKUP: ANSWER: B

(Taveras & Ferrucci, vol 2, chap 109. Amplatz, pp 280, 355-369.) The anteroposterior chest radiograph in complete transposition of the great vessels (TOGV) reveals a narrow mediastinal shadow, created by the overlap of the aorta and pulmonary artery, and an ovoid, malpositioned heart. This appearance has been described as the "egg on its side" or "egg on a string."

In the rarer instance, when the transposition has been congenitally "corrected" by the additional anomaly of ventricular inversion, the heart shape becomes distinctive. The left heart border assumes a boxlike configuration formed by the straight lateral edge of the ascending aorta. The right pulmonary hilum is displaced medially and elevated, producing the "waterfall" appearance. Although this sign was described in reference to this specific entity, it may be seen with other anomalies that have a VSD and high pulmonary blood flow.

The "gooseneck" deformity that is seen with endocardial cushion defects results from the apparent elongation and narrowing of the left ventricular outflow tract that occurs from the deficiencies in the ventricular septum and a cleft in the anterior leaflet of the mitral valve.

193. CLINICAL THERAPEUTICS: CONTINUED CARE: ANSWER: G
194. CLINICAL THERAPEUTICS: CONTINUED CARE: ANSWER: A
195. CLINICAL THERAPEUTICS: CONTINUED CARE: ANSWER: F

(DiSaia, 4/e, pp 376-381.) Bleomycin and doxorubicin are antibiotics whose side effects are pulmonary fibrosis and cardiac toxicity, respectively. Vincristine arrests cells in metaphase by binding microtubular proteins and preventing the formation of mitotic spindles. Peripheral neuropathy is a common side effect.

196. CLINICAL THERAPEUTICS: CONTINUED CARE: ANSWER: C
197. CLINICAL THERAPEUTICS: CONTINUED CARE: ANSWERS: A, D, E, F
198. CLINICAL INTERVENTION: INITIAL WORKUP: ANSWERS: G, I

(Isselbacher, 13/e, pp 1266-1268.) Certain drugs will interfere with the body's compensation of a renal hypoperfusion state, renal artery stenosis, and induce a prerenal azotemia. These drugs include ACE inhibitors and prostaglandin synthesis inhibitors (cyclooxygenase inhibitors). Hepatorenal syndrome occurs when renal failure complicates a preexisting hepatic disease such as cirrhosis. Additionally, the concurrent hypoalbuminemia of cirrhosis contributes to a decrease in intravascular volume as fluid accumulates in extravascular compartments and causes prerenal azotemia. This third spacing also occurs with severe burns, sepsis, and pancreatitis and causes a prerenal azotemia. Gentamycin toxicity results in damage to the proximal tubule and is an intrarenal cause of azotemia. Obstruction of these tubules by filtered light chain proteins (myeloma) or by myoglobin/hemoglobin (crush injury) are renal causes of azotemia. Methicillin can cause an allergic interstitial nephritis and subsequent renal azotemia. This often will resolve with discontinuation of the drug. A straddle injury could result in a urethral injury and subsequent stricture, an example of a postrenal obstruction causing azotemia. Obstruction of the ureters by retroperitoneal fibrosis also will result in postrenal azotemia.

199. CLINICAL INTERVENTION: CONTINUED CARE: ANSWERS: B, C, F, G, H
200. CLINICAL INTERVENTION: CONTINUED CARE: ANSWERS: B, D, E, F, H, I

(Isselbacher, 13/e, pp 1403-1416.) Ulcerative colitis usually presents as an inflammatory process involving the mucosal surface of the colon. The involved segment of the colon typically extends from the rectum proximally in a continuous and uniform fashion. Because of the increased risk of adenocarcinoma of the colon in chronic ulcerative colitis, a prophylactic colectomy should be considered in patients with extensive disease unresponsive to medical management or in patients who develop dysplastic changes in the mucosa detected with barium enema or endoscopy. Fistulae are rare in ulcerative colitis as opposed to in Crohn's disease where fistulae are common and occur between the diseased bowel and adjacent organs, bowel, bladder, vagina, or skin. Both Crohn's disease and ulcerative colitis have increased incidence in whites and Jews in particular, and both are associated with biliary tract disease, especially sclerosing cholangitis. The association with biliary tract disease is stronger in ulcerative colitis than in Crohn's disease. Crohn's disease is a transmural, often granulomatous inflammatory process involving any portion of the GI tract. Involvement is discontinuous and frequently occurs in the terminal ileum and perirectal region. Benign pneumoperitoneum can occur following an air contrast barium enema in patients and is not a typical feature of either disease.

Book B

Correct Answers

Number of items: 200

201. CLINICAL INTERVENTION: EMERGENCY: ANSWER: B
(Isselbacher, 13/e, pp 1194-1197.) Lung infection is quite common in cystic fibrosis patients and often is associated with small volume hemoptysis. Larger volume hemoptysis is usually the result of cor pulmonale with hypertrophy of the bronchial arteries. Transcatheter embolization is an appropriate therapy for such bleeding and can be life-saving. Dual drug regimens are used for pulmonary infections in cystic fibrosis to decrease the development of drug resistant strains. Only 10 percent of patients with cystic fibrosis present with meconium ileus as a neonate. The development of digital clubbing is a nearly universal finding in long-standing cystic fibrosis.

202. CLINICAL INTERVENTION: EMERGENCY: ANSWER: B
(Schwartz, 6/e, pp 1701-1702.) Intussusception is the result of invagination of a segment of bowel into distal bowel lumen. The most common type is ileocolic, which typically appears as a "coiled spring" on barium enema. Ileoileal and colocolic intussusceptions occur less commonly and are not easily diagnosed on barium enema. If bloody mucus, peritonitis, or systemic toxicity have not developed, hydrostatic reduction by barium enema is the appropriate initial treatment. Most patients are successfully managed this way and do not require surgical intervention. Immediate treatment should be instituted to avert the danger of bowel infarction. Recurrence is surprisingly uncommon after either surgical or nonsurgical treatment.

203. DIAGNOSIS: CONTINUED CARE: ANSWER: B
(Isselbacher, 13/e, pp 258-260.) Both the arterial pH and the P_{CO_2} are elevated in the patient presented in the question; the disturbance is alkalosis with hypoventilation. The P_{CO_2} typically increases by 0.5 to 1.0 torr for each meq/L increase in serum bicarbonate. These findings suggest that the hypoventilation is compensatory rather than a primary phenomenon. This assumption is further supported by the absence of clinical lung disease.

204. CLINICAL THERAPEUTICS: CONTINUED CARE: ANSWER: C
(Isselbacher, 13/e, pp 258-260.) The development of a clinically significant metabolic alkalosis in a patient requires not only the loss of acid or addition of alkali, but renal responses that *maintain* the alkalosis. The normal kidney can tremendously augment its excretion of acid or alkali in response to changes in ingested load. However, in the presence of significant volume depletion and consequent avid salt and water retention, the tubular maximum for bicarbonate reabsorption is increased. Correction of volume depletion alone is usually sufficient to correct the alkalosis, since the kidney will then excrete the excess bicarbonate. HCl infusion is usually unnecessary and can be dangerous. Acetazolamide is unlikely to be effective in the face of distal Na^+ reabsorption (in exchange for H^+ secretion). Moreover, to the extent that acetazolamide causes natriuresis, it will exacerbate the volume depletion.

205. CLINICAL INTERVENTION: CONTINUED CARE: ANSWER: D
(*Becker, pp 661-665. Evans, pp 404-405.*) The adrenogenital syndrome due to 21-hydroxylase deficiency is the most frequent cause of sexual ambiguity and the most frequent endocrine cause of neonatal death. Serum 17-hydroxyprogesterone and urinary pregnanetriol are elevated. Neonatal complications are related to salt loss because of inadequate mineralocorticoid production in some of these infants.

206. CLINICAL THERAPEUTICS: CONTINUED CARE: ANSWER: E
(Isselbacher, 13/e, chap 238.) In the first week after renal transplantation, the differential diagnosis of graft dysfunction includes early rejection, hypovolemia, cyclosporine intoxication, acute tubular necrosis, urinary obstruction, and renal artery thrombosis. Cyclosporine can mask many of the classic signs of rejection, such as fever and graft tenderness; renal biopsy is often needed to make the diagnosis. However, renal ultrasonography should precede any manipulation to rule out mechanical outflow obstruction, as it should in any patient with acute deterioration of renal function.

207. HISTORY AND PHYSICAL: INITIAL WORKUP: ANSWER: C
(*Isselbacher, 13/e, p 1338.*) Hematuria is the most common presenting symptom occurring in 75 percent of patients with bladder carcinoma. Squamous cell carcinoma is associated with schistisomiasis and thus is common in the Nile region. Mixed histology suggests carcinoma of the urachal remnant which arises off the bladder dome.

208. DIAGNOSIS: CONTINUED CARE: ANSWER: E
(*Armstrong, pp 407-411.)* Although sarcoidosis, bilateral bronchogenic cancer, echinococcal disease, or Wegener granulomatosis could conceivably result in the widespread pulmonary abnormalities in the figure, only progressive massive fibrosis (PMF) characteristically produces large, ill-defined mid-upper-lung-zone masses bilaterally. PMF is most often associated with coal worker's pneumoconiosis and is related to the quantity of dust exposure. PMF usually starts in the lung periphery, slowly enlarges, and migrates centrally. A helpful differential characteristic of PMF is the tendency for the lesion to have a transverse diameter which is much larger than its anteroposterior diameter. Mortality is due to the severe emphysema which usually accompanies the condition.

209. DIAGNOSIS: CONTINUED CARE: ANSWER: E
(Isselbacher, 13/e, chap 285.) Persons who have rheumatoid arthritis can develop popliteal cysts as a complication of synovitis of the knee. Popliteal cysts can expand upward into the thigh or downward into the calf. Rupture of a popliteal cyst produces sudden pain and swelling; because these symptoms resemble those of thrombophlebitis—though perhaps more dramatic in onset—an arthrogram may be needed to confirm the diagnosis. Although rupture of the plantaris tendon can occur in persons exposed to mechanical trauma, it would not be the most likely diagnosis for the woman described in the question. The anserine bursa is located on the medial aspect of the knee joint and not in the calf. Achilles tendonitis should not cause pain and swelling of the calf.

210. CLINICAL THERAPEUTICS: CONTINUED CARE: ANSWER: B
(Isselbacher, 13/e, chap 227.) A solitary lung nodule in a middle-aged person who is a cigarette smoker requires surgical resection. Although a rheumatoid nodule would be in the differential diagnosis of the lesion described in the case, such nodules are usually subpleural and are more common in men than in women. The central location and small size of the lesion described make it relatively inaccessible to nonsurgical biopsy techniques. Because 95 percent of malignant solitary nodules originate in the lung, an undirected search for a primary source is likely to be fruitless. Mediastinoscopy has largely replaced scalene node biopsy in most centers, but because the incidence of mediastinal metastases in malignant solitary nodules is less than 10 percent, surgical exploration would be indicated for the man described in the question.

211. CLINICAL INTERVENTION: INITIAL WORKUP: ANSWER: E
(Isselbacher, 13/e, chap 384.) This patient displays the characteristic heliotropic rash, with knuckle involvement and proximal muscle weakness typical of dermatomyositis. Although a biopsy could be done, the disease is patchy and the absence of a lymphocytic infiltration would not rule out the diagnosis. EMG will be diagnostic in about 40 percent of affected persons. Since the diagnosis is straightforward and dermatomyositis is frequently associated with malignancy in those over age 60, it is quite reasonable to screen for cancer. In addition to the common epithelial malignancies, myeloproliferative disorders can be heralded by dermatomyositis. However, an unfocused radiological diagnostic attack should definitely be suspended in favor of the simple and cost-effective tests outlined in Choice E. Although steroids will probably be symptomatically beneficial even in those with malignancies, their use should probably be delayed until the screening is completed. If an early neoplasm can be found and treated, the dermatomyositis could respond without the need of resorting to the dangers of high-dose glucocorticoid therapy.

212. CLINICAL INTERVENTION: CONTINUED CARE: ANSWER: B
(Isselbacher, 13/e, chaps 250, 253.) The x-ray presented shows a large malignant-appearing gastric ulcer on the lesser curvature of the stomach. Because the differentiation between benign and malignant gastric ulcer by x-ray is not infallible (there are as many as 25 percent false positives and negatives), the diagnosis of gastric cancer should be confirmed by fiberoptic gastroscopy with brush cytology and at least six biopsies from the ulcer margin. Gastroscopy is useful in diagnosing primary gastric lymphoma, which is associated with a much better 5-year survival rate than is adenocarcinoma. Double-contrast radiographic techniques help to detect small lesions by improving mucosal detail but do not generally improve accuracy in distinguishing benign from malignant ulcers.

213. DIAGNOSTIC STUDIES: CONTINUED CARE: ANSWER: E
(Speroff, 4/e, pp 173-174.) Although menopause occurs most commonly between 48 and 55 years of age, the frequency of ovulation decreases after 40 years of age as ovarian function wanes. Early signs of this climacteric stage relate to the rate of estrogen loss. Dysfunctional uterine bleeding and minimal vasomotor reactions occur commonly when estrogen loss is slow. Patients often have regular periods despite lower estradiol levels, but the cycle shortens primarily from the shortening of the follicular phase. Serum FSH levels may reach postmenopausal levels (greater than 40 mIU/mL) despite this menstrual bleeding, even though LH levels remain in the normal range. The elevated FSH levels indicate a significant reduction in the total number of remaining follicles, with those remaining having less ability to produce estrogen. Ovulation is uncommon, and corpus luteum formation and function are infrequent. Irregular cycles and unpredictable vaginal bleeding are common. Menopausal levels of serum gonadotropins reach a maximum within 1 to 3 years, with the FSH increased tenfold and LH increased threefold over levels during normal ovarian function.

214. APPLYING BASIC CONCEPTS: CONTINUED CARE: ANSWER: E
(Isselbacher, 13/e, p 2382.) All of the choices are causes of muscle wasting associated with neoplasia.

215. APPLYING BASIC CONCEPTS: INITIAL WORKUP: ANSWER: B
(*Herbst, 2/e, pp 93-95.*) Luteinizing hormone (LH) and follicle-stimulating hormone (FSH) are synthesized, stored, and secreted from the basophilic cells of the adenohypophysis (anterior pituitary). It appears that a single cell type makes both LH and FSH.

216. APPLYING BASIC CONCEPTS: INITIAL WORKUP: ANSWER: E
(Schwartz, 5/e, pp 1347-1349.) The liver is second only to regional lymph nodes as a site for metastatic spread of tumors. This is the most common form of hepatic malignancy, with the relative ratio of secondary to primary neoplasms being about 20:1. About 25 to 50 percent of all patients dying of cancer have hepatic metastases at autopsy. The incidence of hepatoma or primary hepatocellular carcinoma is relatively rare in populations from North America and Western Europe, although it is common in certain parts of Africa where primary liver cancer represents 17 to 53 percent of all cancers. Angiosarcoma rarely occurs in the liver, though when it does it has been associated with exposure to vinyl chloride. Hamartomas and hemangiomas are fairly common benign neoplasms of the liver.

217. APPLYING BASIC CONCEPTS: EMERGENCY: ANSWER: E
(Schwartz, 6/e, pp 175-219. Shires, 3/e, pp 291-340. Walt, 3/e, pp 142-159.) The diagnosis of injuries resulting from blunt abdominal trauma is difficult; injuries often are masked by associated injuries. Thus, trauma to the head or chest, together with fractures, frequently conceals intraabdominal injury. Apparently trivial injuries may rupture abdominal viscera in spite of the protection offered by the rib cage. The structures most likely to be damaged in blunt abdominal trauma are, in order of frequency, spleen, kidney, intestine, liver, abdominal wall, mesentery, pancreas, and diaphragm. Abdominal paracentesis is a rapid, sensitive diagnostic test for patients with suspected intraabdominal injury and may be extremely helpful in the management of patients with associated head, thoracic, or pelvic trauma in whom signs and symptoms of the abdominal injuries may be masked or overlooked. Abdominal CT scans, which should be done promptly and rapidly, are being used more frequently to evaluate these injuries.

218. CLINICAL INTERVENTION: EMERGENCY: ANSWER: D
(Schwartz, 5/e, pp 271-273.) The spleen should be salvaged in children if at all possible because of the postsplenectomy septicemia seen at a significantly increased rate in this group. The organisms responsible are most frequently *Diplococcus pneumoniae* and *Haemophilus influenzae*. The most effective method of spleen salvage is via suture repair of the injured segment (splenorrhaphy).

219. HEALTH MAINTENANCE: INITIAL WORKUP: ANSWER: E
(Isselbacher, 13/e, chaps 21, 382.) Fasciculations may occur in a variety of metabolic and toxic disorders, including amyotrophic lateral sclerosis, progressive bulbar palsy, ruptured intervertebral disk, and peripheral neuropathy. However, they should not be viewed with alarm in the absence of weakness, muscle atrophy, or loss of tendon reflexes. The best treatment a physician could offer a person who is asymptomatic except for fascicular twitches is reassurance and, if appropriate, advice to reduce coffee intake.

220. DIAGNOSIS: CONTINUED CARE: ANSWER: C
(Droegemueller, p 824.) Intravenous leiomyomatosis is a benign condition involving the spread of smooth muscle cells from within the myometrium to distant organs such as the lungs. Cells that are stained blue within the lymphatics are suggestive of endolymphatic stromal myosis. The finding of subperitoneal nodules is suggestive of leiomyomatosis peritonealis disseminata.

221. DIAGNOSIS: CONTINUED CARE: ANSWER: E
(Isselbacher, 13/e, chap 368. Fisher, Neurology 32:871, 1982.) A pure motor hemiparesis on one side (with ipsilateral face and body involvement) and no other cortical deficits (aphasia or cortical sensory loss) suggests an internal capsular lesion. The major differential diagnosis in this setting is between a hypertensive hemorrhage or an internal capsular lacunar infarct. Both entities may present with a fluctuating course over hours; however, hemorrhages tend to produce some manifestation of increased intracranial pressure. Lacunar infarctions result from atherothrombotic and hyalinization changes in the penetrating branches of the circle of Willis, middle cerebral artery stem, and vertebrobasilar system. Other than the internal capsule, common locations for lacunar infarctions include the thalamus, where they produce pure sensory deficit, and the base of the pons, where they produce hemiparesis and dysarthria with a clumsy hand. CT scanning can document most supratentorial lacunar infarctions, whose size usually ranges from 0.5 to 2 cm.

222. APPLYING BASIC CONCEPTS: CONTINUED CARE: ANSWER: B
(Isselbacher, 13/e, chap 386.) More than three-quarters of patients with myasthenia have circulating antibodies against components of the postsynaptic membrane, including acetylcholine receptors. Antibody action leads to an unfolding, or "simplification," of the membrane and, consequently, a reduced number of acetylcholine receptors. As a result, existing acetylcholine in the synapse is less effective in producing muscle contraction.

223. PROGNOSIS: CONTINUED CARE: ANSWER: B
(Schwartz, 5/e, pp 1335-1336.) All conditions listed in the question may result in pyogenic liver abscess. Although, in the past, appendicitis was the principal cause, cholangitis is currently the most likely cause. Treatment consists of surgical or percutaneous catheter drainage. For the patient with a large solitary abscess, which is properly drained, the prognosis is good. There remains, however, a substantial mortality associated with multiple abscess formation.

224. HISTORY AND PHYSICAL: INITIAL WORKUP: ANSWER: A
(Isselbacher, 13/e, chap 383.) Entrapment of the lateral femoral cutaneous nerve, which can occur where it enters the thigh beneath the inguinal ligament near the anterior superior iliac spine, causes a sensory neuropathy known as "meralgia paresthetica." Symptoms of this disorder, which typically occur in obese persons, include pain and decreased tactile sensation over the lateral aspect of the thigh. Treatment is infiltration with a local anesthetic or, if this procedure proves ineffective, surgical sectioning of the nerve.

225. DIAGNOSIS: EMERGENCY: ANSWER: D
(Isselbacher, 13/e, chap 383.) The inflammatory response in Guillain-Barré syndrome strips myelin between the nodes of Ranvier in peripheral nerves. This phenomenon explains both the slowing of nerve conduction and the potential for recovery. Axons are only destroyed in extensively involved areas as a secondary phenomenon. To date, no convincing evidence has emerged to support the contention that the central nervous system is involved in Guillain-Barré syndrome.

226. PROGNOSIS: CONTINUED CARE: ANSWER: E
(*Isselbacher, 13/e, p 2372.*) Eighty-five percent of patients with Guillain-Barré syndrome recover fully or nearly so. Two-thirds of cases are triggered by a preceding viral syndrome, most often due to a

herpesvirus (CMV or EBV). Immunoglobulin treatment is likely as effective as plasmapheresis and can be beneficial if given in the first two weeks of the illness. Treatment with glucocorticoids has not been shown to be effective in Guillain-Barré syndrome. One third of patients with Guillain-Barré syndrome will require ventilatory support and 5 percent will die from the disease.

227. HISTORY AND PHYSICAL: INITIAL WORKUP: ANSWER: E
(Schwartz, 6/e, pp 1509-1511.) Idiopathic retroperitoneal fibrosis is a nonsuppurative inflammatory process of the retroperitoneum that causes problems by extrinsic compression of retroperitoneal structures. The ureters, aorta, and inferior vena cava are most at risk; however, the aorta is quite resistant to compression and the inferior vena cava has multiple collaterals so that ureteral obstruction is the most common presentation of this disease process. The common bile duct and duodenum may be compressed and obstructed, but this occurs much less frequently. Treatment of ureteral obstruction includes conservative therapy with steroids. Often surgical intervention is required and ureterolysis with intraperitoneal transplantation is the current procedure of choice. Biopsies must also be taken to exclude a malignant process as the cause of the fibrosis.

228. DIAGNOSIS: INITIAL WORKUP: ANSWER: D
(Sabiston and Spencer, 5/e, pp 1901-1919. Schwartz, 5/e, pp 882-883.) The patient described in the question manifests evidence of heart disease, a finding that is uncommonly associated with cardiac tumors other than myxomas. Myxomas are the most common primary cardiac tumors, constituting approximately half the primary tumors of the heart. Sarcomas account for about a quarter. Other primary tumors, such as hemangiomas and rhabdomyomas, are extremely rare. Malignant lymphoma and metastatic carcinoma, although usually asymptomatic and seldom seen except at autopsy, represent the most common of all cardiac neoplasms. Myxoma is a benign polypoid tumor that usually affects the left atrium. Because of its size, form, and location, the tumor compromises intracardiac blood flow and can mimic many primary cardiac diseases. While it does not invade contiguous structures nor does it metastasize, myxoma does tend to fragment and embolize. Hence, in atypical cases of acute arterial occlusion, such as in asymptomatic young patients who do not have a history of cardiac disease, histologic examination of emboli should be performed to rule out myxoma.

229. DIAGNOSTIC STUDIES: CONTINUED CARE: ANSWER: A
(Isselbacher, 13/e, chap 377.) Acquired hepatocerebral degeneration is a neurologic syndrome composed mainly of extrapyramidal signs. A well-known consequence of chronic liver disease, this disorder simulates Wilson's disease in many ways, including the presence of neuropathologic lesions in the cortex, basal ganglia, and other deep nuclei. Many cases become evident after a bout of hepatic encephalopathy, but others occur insidiously in persons who never have had encephalopathy.

230. DIAGNOSTIC STUDIES: CONTINUED CARE: ANSWER: C
(Isselbacher, 13/e, p 1441.) An MRI will evaluate the two most common causes of major motor aphasia—posterior frontal lobe mass lesions and emboli in the superior branch of the left middle cerebral artery. Cranial CT will not be as sensitive to this latter abnormality. Plain films of the skull and mastoid air cells and brain scanning are insensitive and not indicated. Conventional angiography can demonstrate frontal lobe lesions and embolic changes in the middle cerebral artery, but has been replaced by magnetic resonance angiography because of its decreased risk, cost, and morbidity for screening evaluation of the major intracranial vessels.

231. DIAGNOSIS: EMERGENCY: ANSWER: A
(Isselbacher, 13/e, chaps 374, 381.) Spinal epidural abscess, a neurologic emergency, is currently best diagnosed by MRI. Lumbar puncture would show a high protein content and cell count but would not establish the diagnosis and may in fact be harmful. Babinski signs are absent in the case described because lumbar pain indicates an abscess overlying the cauda equina, which is made up of peripheral nerves, rather than the spinal cord.

232. DIAGNOSIS: INITIAL WORKUP: ANSWER: B
(Isselbacher, 13/e, chap 18.) The symptoms and signs described in the question are most consistent with Ménière's disease. In this disorder, paroxysmal vertigo due to labyrinthine lesions is associated with nausea, vomiting, rotatory nystagmus, tinnitus, high-tone hearing loss with recruitment, and, most characteristically, fullness in the ear. Labyrinthitis would be an unlikely diagnosis in the case presented because of the hearing loss and multiple episodes. Vertebral-basilar insufficiency and multiple sclerosis typically are associated with brainstem signs. Acoustic neuroma only rarely causes vertigo as its initial symptom, and the vertigo it causes is mild and intermittent.

233. CLINICAL INTERVENTION: EMERGENCY: ANSWER: D
(Isselbacher, 13/e, chap 197.) Sinus bradycardia and a long sinus pause raise the possibility of sick sinus syndrome, which is not an infrequent cause of lightheadedness among the elderly. It is important that the relationship between symptoms and the arrhythmias documented by Holter monitoring be clarified before implantation of a permanent pacemaker is considered. An exercise tolerance test, though it may strengthen the suspicion of sick sinus syndrome by showing an inadequate heart rate response, cannot prove that the condition is responsible for the patient's symptoms. Sublingual isoproterenol has little usefulness in the management of chronic bradyarrhythmias.

234. CLINICAL INTERVENTION: CONTINUED CARE: ANSWER: B
(Isselbacher, 13/e, chap 198.) The rhythm demonstrated in the electrocardiogram presented is multifocal atrial tachycardia, which is characterized by variable P-wave morphology and PR and RR intervals. Control of multifocal atrial tachycardia, usually associated with severe pulmonary disease, comes with improved ventilation and oxygenation. Carotid sinus massage, electrical cardioversion, and administration of digitalis, verapamil, or quinidine are of little benefit, although verapamil may temporarily slow the ventricular rate.

235. CLINICAL INTERVENTION: CONTINUED CARE: ANSWER: E
(*Reece, p 832.*) Numerous changes occur in the cardiovascular system during pregnancy. Heart rate increases about 10 to 15 beats per minute. Blood volume and cardiac output increase significantly. Many cardiac sounds that would be abnormal in a nonpregnant state are normal during pregnancy. All the findings listed in the question are normal. Ninety percent of pregnant women will have systolic ejection murmurs. In approximately 20 percent of women, a soft diastolic murmur can be heard.

236. DIAGNOSIS: INITIAL WORKUP: ANSWER: E
(Isselbacher, 13/e, chap 371, 379.) The combination of autonomic insufficiency and parkinsonian symptoms is known as the Shy-Drager syndrome. The autonomic form of the Landry-Guillain-Barré syndrome causes acute autonomic paralysis but does not cause the parkinsonian symptoms of tremor at rest, bradykinesia, and rigidity. A number of antihypertensive agents cause orthostatic hypotension, but

none cause parkinsonism. Micturition syncope is a condition in which syncope occurs because of vagal surge at the time of release of intravesicular pressure.

237. APPLYING BASIC CONCEPTS: EMERGENCY: ANSWER: D
(Isselbacher, 13/e, chap 368.) Half of all episodes of hypertensive intracerebral hemorrhage occur in the putamen and the adjacent internal capsule. Other sites, in decreasing order of frequency, are the thalamus, cerebellar hemispheres, and pons. Hemorrhages in the subcortical white matter are not generally associated with hypertension and should prompt a search for a bleeding diathesis or an underlying brain lesion. The diagnosis of brain hemorrhage is suggested by clinical signs and confirmed by CT scan; lumbar puncture no longer is recommended.

238. DIAGNOSTIC STUDIES: CONTINUED CARE: ANSWER: A
(Isselbacher, 13/e, chap 369. Hochberg, J Neurosurg 68:835, 1988.) Lymphoma of the brain (usually diffuse large cell) is increasingly common as a sporadic tumor and occurs frequently in immunosuppressed patients, especially in those with AIDS. Its clinical sensitivity to corticosteroids can mistakenly suggest a diagnosis of multiple sclerosis, and its complete disappearance or dramatic improvement on CT scan after steroid therapy is baffling. Radiosensitivity is a well-known feature of most primary CNS lymphomas, which are almost always of B-cell origin.

239. PROGNOSIS: CONTINUED CARE: ANSWER: A
(Isselbacher, 13/e, pp 1775-1777.) The initial response to chemotherapy and radiotherapy is striking with partial or complete response in 75 percent of patients. Median survival is just 2 years, however. There is no curative role for surgery in this disease, as it is often multifocal including epidural spinal lesions. The frequency of this lesion is increasing, as immunocompromised patients are susceptible to primary CNS lymphoma, i.e., AIDS patients and post-transplant patients on immunosuppressive, anti-rejection therapy.

240. LEGAL AND ETHICAL ISSUES: EMERGENCY: ANSWER: E
(*Herbst, 2/e, pp 363-368, 373-375.*) Although all the procedures mentioned in the question can be helpful in establishing a case of rape in most situations, the expected lack of sperm and the matching blood types in the situation presented would limit their value in this case. Only the finding of 50 units/mL or more of acid phosphatase in this woman's vagina could be taken as evidence of ejaculation. Her introitus probably would not be injured because of her parity. Foreign pubic hair might only indicate close contact.

241. DIAGNOSIS: EMERGENCY: ANSWER: C
(Schwartz, 5/e, pp 1090-1091.) Blood passed per rectum is caused most often by bleeding that originates in the upper gastrointestinal tract. However, in bleeding that does not originate from lesions distal to the ligament of Trietz, colonic carcinoma is the most common cause of bloody stools. Diverticulosis is the most common cause of massive lower gastrointestinal bleeding. Meckel's diverticulum, diverticulitis, and ulcerative colitis are all less common causes of rectal bleeding. When occult or gross blood is found in stools, carcinoma of the colon must be ruled out.

242. HISTORY AND PHYSICAL: EMERGENCY: ANSWER: E
(*Isselbacher, 13/e, p 1121.)* The presence of focal neurologic findings should suggest infarction, hemorrhage, or TIA. Hypertension, usually severe, is a hallmark of hypertensive encephalopathy.

243. DIAGNOSIS: INITIAL WORKUP: ANSWER: E
(Isselbacher, 13/e, chap 358.) The combination of hypocalcemia, hypophosphatemia, elevated serum parathyroid hormone levels, and bone fractures is consistent with a diagnosis of osteomalacia in this patient. In the absence of other gastrointestinal or renal abnormalities leading to malabsorption or increased renal loss of calcium or phosphorus, vitamin D deficiency is likely to be present. Inadequate intake of vitamin D and calcium together with limited exposure to the sun are frequent in this age group. Postmenopausal osteoporosis is associated with vertebral and hip fractures as well, but laboratory abnormalities are not present. Primary hyperparathyroidism is associated with increased serum calcium concentration, as is ectopic parathyroid hormone secretion (although existence of the latter has been questioned). Paget's disease of the bone does not produce hypocalcemia, and it causes typical sclerotic changes on x-ray examination.

244. DIAGNOSIS: INITIAL WORKUP: ANSWER: D
(*Carr, pp 60-63.*) In North America, any pubertal changes before the age of 8 years in girls and 9 years in boys are regarded as precocious. Although the most common type of precocious puberty in girls is idiopathic, it is essential to ensure close long-term follow-up of these patients to ascertain that there is not serious underlying pathology, such as tumors of the central nervous system or ovary. Only 1 to 2 percent of patients with precocious puberty have an estrogen-producing ovarian tumor as the causative factor. McCune-Albright syndrome (polyostotic fibrous dysplasia) is also relatively rare and consists of fibrous dysplasia and cystic degeneration of the long bones, sexual precocity, and café au lait spots on the skin. Hypothyroidism is a cause of precocious puberty in some children, making thyroid function tests mandatory in these cases. Tumors of the central nervous system as a cause of precocious puberty occur more commonly in boys than in girls; they are seen in about 11 percent of girls with precocious puberty.

245. CLINICAL THERAPEUTICS: CONTINUED CARE: ANSWER: B
(Isselbacher, 13/e, chap 367.) Absence, or petit mal, seizures are distinguished from complex partial seizures in a number of ways, including lack of an aura, a characteristic 3-Hz rhythmic EEG pattern during a spell, and immediate recovery. Because of their brevity and subtlety, absence seizures frequently go unrecognized until an affected child begins school and performs poorly. The prognosis is good: one-third outgrow the disorder, one-third have a milder form in adulthood, and one-third have easily controlled generalized seizures. Ethosuximide and valproic acid, not phenytoin, are the drugs of choice.

246. DIAGNOSIS: INITIAL WORKUP: ANSWER: D
(Isselbacher, 13/e, chap 361.) Paget's disease of the bone is relatively common, and the incidence increases with age. An estimated prevalence of 3 percent in persons over the age of 40 years is a generally accepted figure. Most frequently, the disease is asymptomatic and diagnosed only when the typical sclerotic bones are incidentally detected on x-ray examinations done for other reasons or when an increased alkaline phosphatase activity is recognized on routine laboratory measurements. The etiology is unknown, but increased bone resorption followed by intensive bone repair is thought to be the mechanism causing increased bone density and increased serum alkaline phosphatase activity as a marker of osteoblast activity. Since increased mineralization of bone takes place (although in an abnormal pattern), hypercalcemia is not present unless a severely affected patient becomes immobilized. Hypercalcemia, in fact, would be an expected finding in a patient with primary hyperparathyroidism,

bone metastases, or plasmacytoma, the last typically producing no increase in the alkaline phosphatase activity. Osteomalacia resulting from vitamin D deficiency is associated with bone pain and hypophosphatemia; normal or decreased serum calcium concentration produces secondary hyperparathyroidism, further aggravating the defective bone mineralization.

247. APPLYING BASIC CONCEPTS: INITIAL WORKUP: ANSWER: B
(Isselbacher, 13/e, chap 333.) Patients with lung cancer, particularly small cell carcinoma, frequently present with the syndrome of inappropriate vasopressin (AVP, antidiuretic hormone) secretion. Indeed, more than half of patients with such tumors show evidence of inappropriate secretion of AVP, even when serum sodium concentration remains normal. AVP is produced by the tumor tissue itself and is chemically identical to arginine vasopressin secreted by the neurohypophysis. Central nervous system lesions of infectious, inflammatory, and vascular etiologies can also result in inappropriate AVP secretion, but intracerebral metastases from lung carcinomas are not usually responsible for inappropriate AVP secretion.

248. HISTORY AND PHYSICAL: EMERGENCY: ANSWER: E
(Isselbacher, 13/e, chap 251.) A Zenker's diverticulum typically causes halitosis and regurgitation of saliva and food particles consumed several days earlier. When a Zenker's diverticulum fills with food, it may produce dysphagia by compressing the esophagus. Gastric outlet obstruction can cause bloating and regurgitation of newly ingested food. Gastrointestinal disorders associated with scleroderma include esophageal reflux, the development of wide-mouthed colonic diverticula, and stasis and bacterial overgrowth. Achalasia typically presents with dysphagia for both solids and liquids. Gastric retention caused by the autonomic neuropathy of diabetes mellitus usually results in postprandial epigastric discomfort and bloating.

249. HEALTH MAINTENANCE: INITIAL WORKUP: ANSWER: E
(Isselbacher, 13/e, chap 357.) Because of the ease of screening for hypercalcemia, this is now the most frequent presentation of hyperparathyroidism. This early, pre-symptomatic diagnosis has reduced the end-organ damage seen in hyperparathyroidism, particularly reducing nephrolithiasis and bone involvement. Parathormone acts directly on the kidney to increase urinary phosphate excretion and thus lowers serum phosphate levels. Most cases of primary hyperparathyroidism are sporadic and due to an adenoma; however, a strong family history of hyperparathyroidism suggests a multiple endocrine neoplasia syndrome. Often the adenoma is not localized pre-operatively and careful surgical technique and immediate pathologic confirmation of the excised parathyroid glands are required.

250. LEGAL AND ETHICAL ISSUES: INITIAL WORKUP: ANSWER: E
(Herbst, 2/e, pp 192-198.) Studies on adult sexual behavior have shown that it is the result of interactions of biologic, psychologic, developmental, and sociologic factors. Studies on lesbian women have been non-diagnostic in terms of finding either altered hormonal states or altered personality traits from other women. In separate surveys, 49 percent of lesbians stated "yes" they did consider having children, and the same number stated that they told their physicians of their lesbianism. Of those lesbians who did not inform their doctors of this fact, most stated that they did not because of fear of jeopardizing their medical care.

251. PROGNOSIS: CONTINUED CARE: ANSWER: A

(Sabiston and Spencer, 5/e, pp 503-504. Schwartz, 6/e, pp 921-922.) Superior vena cava obstruction is almost always due to malignancy and, in three out of four cases, results from invasion of the vena cava by bronchogenic carcinoma. Lymphomas account for most of the remaining cases of the superior vena cava syndrome. Fibrosing mediastinitis as a complication of histoplasmosis or ingestion of methysergide may occur but is rare. Rarely a substernal thyroid or thoracic aortic aneurysm may be responsible for the obstruction. Although constrictive pericarditis may decrease venous return to the heart, it does not produce obstruction of the superior vena cava. Whatever the cause of the superior vena cava syndrome, the resultant increased venous pressure produces edema of the upper body, cyanosis, dilated subcutaneous collateral vessels in the chest, and headache. Cervical lymphadenopathy may also be present as a result of either stasis or metastatic involvement. When carcinoma is the cause of the superior vena cava syndrome, the treatment is usually palliative and consists of diuretics and radiation.

252. CLINICAL INTERVENTION: INITIAL WORKUP: ANSWER: A

(Isselbacher, 13/e, chaps 48, 340.) In a 7-year-old girl, isosexual precocity that is associated with undetectable levels of gonadotropins and urinary 17-ketosteroid levels appropriate for her chronologic age is most likely due to an estrogen-secreting tumor. Tumor localization procedures, such as abdominal CT scanning and pelvic sonography, should be performed before laparotomy. Plasma androstenedione measurement is unlikely to be helpful if urinary 17-ketosteroid excretion is low or normal. In idiopathic precocious puberty, a diagnosis of exclusion, urinary gonadotropins are either normal for chronologic age or elevated; in addition, if plasma gonadotropins are measured frequently during a 24-h period, the characteristic pubertal nocturnal surge should be seen in patients with idiopathic precocious puberty.

253. DIAGNOSIS: CONTINUED CARE: ANSWER: C

(Isselbacher, 13/e, pp 1679-1684.) Sarcoidosis typically occurs in young, black females and often presents mainly with pulmonary symptoms. Hypercalcemia occurs in 1 to 2 percent of patients and can result in nephrolithiasis. Renal infarctions are very rare and are not a feature of sarcoidosis. The history is not compatible with Wegener's granulomatosis, which is rare in blacks. Pulmonary symptoms are common including cough, dyspnea, and chest pain. Treatment consists of cyclophosphamide. The patient's age and sex support the diagnosis of primary pulmonary hypertension, PPH, as does her dyspnea. The nodular skin lesions of sarcoidosis, erythema nodosum, are not associated with PPH or reactive airway disease, nor is renal involvement.

254. HEALTH MAINTENANCE: INITIAL WORKUP: ANSWER: B

(*Isselbacher, 13/e, pp 1324-1326.*) The patient has autosomal dominant polycystic kidney disease. This disorder usually presents in the third or fourth decade with hypertension and flank fullness or pain. Urine output is maintained and fluid overload is not a clinical feature of this disease. The imaging findings described and the strong family history are sufficient for the diagnosis to be made. Ten percent of patients affected with autosomal dominant polycystic kidney disease will have neurologic symptoms from bleeding berry aneurysms at some point during their lifetime, but routine screening angiography is not indicated. Screening of the patient's children is recommended given the autosomal dominant inheritance pattern of this disease.

255. CLINICAL INTERVENTION: CONTINUED CARE: ANSWER: C
(Isselbacher, 13/e, chap 265.) Benign postoperative intrahepatic cholestasis can develop as a consequence of major surgery for a catastrophic event in which hypotension, extensive blood loss into tissues, and massive blood replacement are notable. Factors contributing to jaundice include the pigment load from transfusions, decreased liver function due to hypotension, and decreased renal bilirubin excretion due to tubular necrosis. Jaundice becomes evident on the second or third postoperative day, with bilirubin levels (mainly levels of conjugated bilirubin) peaking by the tenth day. Serum alkaline phosphatase concentration may be elevated up to tenfold, but aspartate aminotransferase (AST) levels are only mildly elevated. Hepatitis and hepatic infarct are unlikely diagnoses in the absence of abdominal pain or tenderness or a significant rise in AST levels. The incubation period of posttransfusion hepatitis is 7 weeks, making this diagnosis unlikely.

256. APPLYING BASIC CONCEPTS: INITIAL WORKUP: ANSWER: B
(Sabiston and Spencer, 5/e, pp 560, 573-574.) Pancoast's tumors are peripheral bronchogenic carcinomas that produce symptoms by involvement of extrapulmonary structures adjacent to the cupula. These structures include the nerve roots of C8 and T1, as well as the sympathetic trunk. Interruption of the cervical sympathetic trunk leads to miosis, ptosis, and anhidrosis, the triad of signs that constitutes Horner's syndrome. Involvement of the nerve roots causes pain along the corresponding dermatomes. The peripheral location of the neoplasm makes pulmonary signs, such as atelectasis and cough, unlikely.

257. DIAGNOSTIC STUDIES: CONTINUED CARE: ANSWER: C
(Cunningham, 18/e, pp 599-608.) A delta OD_{450} result in zone II or zone III during the second half of pregnancy suggests ongoing hemolysis of fetal red blood cells because of high absorption of breakdown pigments, mostly bilirubin. Concentrations high in zone II or in zone III are suggestive of a more severely affected infant; a value of 0.3 or greater is associated with fetal death within several days unless early delivery or intrauterine transfusion is attempted. A patient with an initial high value requires a repeat ultrasound examination and amniocentesis unless ultrasound findings already suggest hydropic change. A newer alternative would be cordocentesis with determinations of fetal hematocrit and blood type. Hydrops fetalis involves subcutaneous edema and effusions into serous cavities in severely affected infants. The placenta is usually quite edematous, boggy, and enlarged, with prominent cotyledons. With abnormally high concentrations of bilirubin in the amniotic fluid, intrauterine fetal transfusions between 23 and 32 weeks are necessary. At or beyond 32 weeks of gestation, a nontransfused but severely affected fetus will likely survive if delivered and treated aggressively. Along with gestational age and fetal size at the time of first transfusion, the prognosis is influenced by the development of signs of ascites and pericardial effusions. The subsequent development of children who previously underwent intrauterine transfusion is generally good, but depends on the severity of the hemolysis and the age of gestation at delivery.

258. CLINICAL THERAPEUTICS: CONTINUED CARE: ANSWER: B
(Isselbacher, 13/e, chap 198.) The rhythm strip shows polymorphic ventricular tachycardia characteristic of torsades de pointes ("twisting of the points"). This life-threatening rhythm is associated with prolongation of the QT interval, resulting, in this case, from the administration of quinidine. The appropriate therapy is to discontinue the offending agent and to withhold other agents that prolong the QT interval, such as procainamide. Hypokalemia can also prolong QT interval and result in this rhythm; however, this patient had normal serum electrolyte concentrations.

259. CLINICAL INTERVENTION: EMERGENCY: ANSWER: C

(Isselbacher, 13/e, chap 223.) Certain persons with severe obstructive lung disease appear to respond to uncontrolled oxygen therapy by dangerously reducing their minute ventilation. Because they are relatively insensitive to changes in arterial P_{CO_2}, hypoxemia is the major ventilatory stimulus in these persons. When hypoxemia is suddenly treated with supplemental oxygen therapy given in an uncontrolled fashion, ventilation drops, arterial P_{CO_2} rises, acidosis results, and coma may develop. However, abrupt removal of supplemental oxygen may precipitate life-threatening hypoxemia. Because acidosis must nevertheless be rapidly reversed by increasing ventilation, endotracheal intubation should be performed, followed by mechanical ventilation of sufficient amount to return arterial pH to physiologic range. Inhaled bronchodilators cannot be given to comatose, unintubated persons. Epinephrine is relatively ineffective in persons with acute or chronic respiratory failure and is dangerous in elderly, acidemic patients.

260. CLINICAL THERAPEUTICS: CONTINUED CARE: ANSWER: D

(Isselbacher, 13/e, chap 223.) Right ventricular failure in persons with chronic pulmonary disease is usually evident as edema and ascites—that is, signs of increased extravascular water. Evidence also suggests that increased right ventricular filling pressures contribute to increases in lung water. Treatment should be aimed at reducing the afterload of the right ventricle. This goal can be accomplished most physiologically by increasing alveolar oxygen tension with supplemental oxygen therapy. Although hydralazine and diazoxide are vasodilators with important effects on the pulmonary circulation, they would not be needed in the case described and may, in fact, worsen gas exchange. Although the usefulness of digoxin therapy in cor pulmonale is debated, the drug generally is reserved for treating persons who have coexisting left ventricular disease. Phlebotomy, although it may improve oxygen delivery in persons with right ventricular failure and elevated hemoglobin concentrations (> 200 g/L [20 g/dL]), would not be a reliable remedy for the ascites and edema in the patient presented.

261. CLINICAL THERAPEUTICS: CONTINUED CARE: ANSWER: E

(Isselbacher, 13/e, chap 267.) Glucocorticoid therapy has been shown to prolong survival in patients with chronic active hepatitis of nonviral etiology. This patient, who has evidence of chronic hepatitis B infection as the cause of her chronic active hepatitis (this diagnosis has been made because of piecemeal necrosis on liver biopsy), would not benefit from administration of steroids. Though many agents have been tried in chronic active viral hepatitis, none have thus far been shown to be effective in the majority of patients. Small randomized studies using alpha interferon have shown promise in that improvement in liver histology has been observed.

262. CLINICAL INTERVENTION: CONTINUED CARE: ANSWER: A

(*Isselbacher, 13/e, pp 1655-1659.*) Atrophy and fibrotic replacement in the bowel wall result in dysmotility of the lower two-thirds of the esophagus, wide-mouth sacculations or diverticula in the colon, and pseudoobstruction. The hypomotility can result in malabsorption syndromes which result from bacterial overgrowth. Air in the bowel wall or frank pneumoperitoneum can occur and be asymptomatic and self-limited. These GI manifestations can precede the development of cutaneous lesions.

263. DIAGNOSIS: CONTINUED CARE: ANSWER: D

(Mattingly, 6/e, pp 332-334.) Ureteral injury is a serious complication of hysterectomy. The course of the ureters is in close proximity to the uterus and ovaries, and surgeons performing pelvic procedures

should identify the ureters during the course of dissection. In this way, ureteral injury can either be avoided or diagnosed intraoperatively. The injury most commonly occurs when pelvic anatomy is distorted, as in pelvic inflammatory disease, ovarian cancer, and severe endometriosis. Classically, ureteral injury occurs during a hemorrhage episode, where exposure is lacking and the surgeon may carelessly place clamps in an effort to control bleeding. The most common site of injury is just lateral to the cervix, with the second most common site being posterior to the infundibulopelvic ligament. Patients with an undiagnosed injury to the ureter usually develop a fever and flank pain. Urinary output may not be noticeably decreased unless, of course, bilateral ureteral ligation has occurred. The diagnosis is confirmed by performing an intravenous pyelogram. Ultrasound can identify a urinoma and rule out perinephric abscess. Urinary culture should be obtained, remembering that urinary infection can coexist with ureteral injury. Drainage of urine from the vagina requires the performance of cystoscopy to distinguish vesicovaginal fistula from ureterovaginal fistula.

If a ureteral stent can be placed past an area of ureteral injury, often the damage will heal within several weeks without further intervention; the stent can then be removed. Complete ureteral obstruction requires reoperation with either ureteroneocystostomy or ureteroureterostomy, depending on the site of injury.

264. DIAGNOSTIC STUDIES: CONTINUED CARE: ANSWER: C

(Isselbacher, 13/e, chap 268.) Primary erythrocytosis with organomegaly strongly suggests the diagnosis of polycythemia rubra vera. One well-recognized complication of this condition is hypercoagulability, with a particular propensity toward hepatic vein thrombosis. Such an occlusion would lead to the Budd-Chiari syndrome characterized by a grossly enlarged, tender liver with severe ascites. In addition to hepatic vein thrombosis secondary to a hypercoagulable state, such a syndrome could result from idiopathic causes, hepatic invasion by tumor, or the venoocclusive disease associated with chemotherapy or radiation. Once right-sided heart failure is excluded clinically, the diagnosis is best established by hepatic venography or liver biopsy showing sinusoidal dilatation.

265. CLINICAL INTERVENTION: CONTINUED CARE: ANSWER: A

(Isselbacher, 13/e, chap 256. Trotman, Gut 29:218, 1988.) This presentation is classic for one of the three clinical variants of the irritable bowel syndrome, each associated with abnormal colonic motility. Other groups have chronic abdominal pain and constipation or alternating constipation and diarrhea. The chronic nature of the condition and the presence of formed stool militate against a workup for secretory or osmotic diarrhea. Giardiasis, while typically occult and requiring jejunal sampling for diagnosis, usually presents with belching and pain, not diarrhea of 4 years' duration. The absence of discernible significant organic pathology should not prompt a discussion with the patient that centers on a psychogenic cause of her problem; such an approach will frequently lead to alienation of the patient. Instead, an effort to effect safe symptomatic improvement of the diarrhea with antispasmodics is worthwhile. Psyllium to increase stool bulk is a good choice for patients with irritable bowel syndrome who complain of constipation.

266. PROGNOSIS: CONTINUED CARE: ANSWER: D

(*Isselbacher, 13/e, pp 1466-1470.*) Hepatitis A most commonly is spread via a fecal-oral transmission route. The onset of symptoms is acute and there are virtually never long-term sequelae. There is no association with the development of hepatocellular carcinoma, nor is there a carrier state associated with hepatitis A.

267. PROGNOSIS: CONTINUED CARE: ANSWER: D
(Schwartz, 6/e, pp 1177, 1316.) Carcinoid tumors arise from the neuroectoderm and are a type of apudoma. The most common site of carcinoid tumors is the small bowel, although appendiceal carcinoids are also common. Carcinoid syndrome, which is characterized by flushing, diarrhea, and cardiac valvular disease, occurs in a small percentage of patients with carcinoid tumors; it is rarely seen with appendiceal carcinoids. The appropriate therapy for a small carcinoid (less than 2 cm) of the appendix is simple appendectomy.

268. HISTORY AND PHYSICAL: CONTINUED CARE: ANSWER: A
(*DiSaia, 4/e, pp 334-337.*) Approximately 50 percent of women who have ovarian cancer present with abdominal distention, and 50 percent present with abdominal pain. Gastrointestinal symptoms, which occur in about 20 percent of affected women, often are secondary to the development of ascites. Urinary tract symptoms, caused by the pressure exerted by a rapidly growing mass, and abnormal vaginal bleeding are the initial symptoms of ovarian cancer in 15 percent of affected women.

269. DIAGNOSIS: CONTINUED CARE: ANSWER: D
(Isselbacher, 13/e, chap 275.) Purtscher's retinopathy is a relatively rare but devastating complication of acute pancreatitis. It is characterized by sudden loss of vision and the presence of cotton-wool spots and hemorrhages in the area of the optic disc and macula. The cause is thought to be occlusion of the posterior retinal artery by aggregated granulocytes.

270. CLINICAL THERAPEUTICS: CONTINUED CARE: ANSWER: C
(Berek, pp 533-536. Hacker, p 392.) After hysterectomy, third-spacing of the body fluids can occur, induced by the surgical injury and by peritoneal dehydration. Brisk IV fluid administration during the first 24 h postoperatively will maintain an adequate urinary output despite movement of fluid into the extravascular compartment, intraoperative blood loss, and the patient's NPO status. Thereafter, maintenance (lesser) rates of infusion are appropriate. The body's daily sodium requirement, in the presence of normal kidney function, allows for hypotonic saline infusions; however, with several days of IV infusion rates that exceed the needs of fluid maintenance, hyponatremia may result. This is not usually due to a sodium deficit but rather to an excess of free water; by fluid restriction the serum sodium will normalize. The kidneys have obligate potassium secretion in the distal tubule and, therefore, 20 to 40 meq of potassium is required daily to maintain the serum level within the normal range. Patients who are more critically ill may appropriately be evaluated with urine electrolytes and osmolality determinations.

271. DIAGNOSIS: CONTINUED CARE: ANSWER: D
(Sabiston and Spencer, 5/e, pp 1134-1146.) Coarctation of the aorta is a congenital anomaly that usually causes aortic stenosis just distal to the left subclavian artery in the area of the ligamentum arteriosum. Collateral circulation develops around the obstruction by way of intercostal vessels and accounts for the classic x-ray appearance of rib notching. Without surgery, the average life span is about 30 to 40 years with eventual death from cardiac failure, rupture of aortic aneurysms or of a cerebral artery, and bacterial endocarditis. Surgery can be accomplished with less than a 1 percent mortality and should be performed around 5 years of age, when the aorta is sufficiently large to be operable but before it becomes fibrotic and calcified, conditions that increase the technical difficulty of the operation.

272. CLINICAL INTERVENTION: EMERGENCY: ANSWER: E
(Isselbacher, 13/e, chap 272.) The radiograph reproduced in the question shows emphysematous cholecystitis, a form of acute cholecystitis in which the gallbladder, its wall, and sometimes even the bile ducts contain gas secondary to infection by gas-producing bacteria. This condition occurs most frequently in elderly men and diabetic persons. The morbidity and mortality rates associated with emphysematous cholecystitis exceed those of acute cholecystitis. Once preoperative preparations are complete, laparotomy and cholecystectomy should be performed promptly.

273. CLINICAL INTERVENTION: EMERGENCY: ANSWER: B
(Isselbacher, 13/e, chap 259.) Virtually any condition that can lead to abdominal pain needs to be included in the differential diagnosis of appendicitis. Diagnostic accuracy is about 75 percent. Although acute diverticulitis, cholecystitis, perforated ulcer, pancreatitis, obstruction, renal stone, and pyelonephritis can present diagnostic difficulties, the most frequent findings at operation when appendicitis is incorrectly diagnosed are (in order of frequency) mesenteric lymphadenitis, no organic disease, acute pelvic inflammatory disease, ruptured ovarian cyst, and acute gastroenteritis.

274. CLINICAL THERAPEUTICS: CONTINUED CARE: ANSWER: E
(Isselbacher, 13/e, chap 275.) Conventional therapy for acute pancreatitis includes analgesia, intravenous volume replacement, and abstinence from oral intake to "rest" the pancreas. Controlled trials have not demonstrated any benefit to symptomatic recovery or survival rate by administration of cimetidine, aprotinin (an inhibitor of pancreatic enzyme release), antibiotics, or glucagon. However, antibiotics are beneficial when secondary infection supervenes (e.g., abscess, phlegmon, or ascending cholangitis). Anticholinergic agents have not been shown to be beneficial and may worsen tachycardia, bowel hypomotility, and oliguria.

275. APPLYING BASIC CONCEPTS: INITIAL WORKUP: ANSWER: E
(*Kurman, 3/e, pp 5, 659-660, 686-688.*) Most ovarian neoplasms in children are of germ cell origin, and about half of these tumors are malignant. Functioning ovarian tumors have been reported to produce precocious puberty in about 2 percent of affected patients. Epithelial tumors of the ovary, which are quite rare in prepubertal girls, are benign in approximately 90 percent of all cases.

276. CLINICAL INTERVENTION: CONTINUED CARE: ANSWER: A
(*DiSaia, 4/e, pp 66-70.*) Cervical cancer frequently presents with a watery discharge and postcoital spotting. Surgical staging by the Gynecologic Oncology Group has revealed periaortic node involvement in 5.6 percent of stage I lesions. Five-year survival rates of approximately 90 percent are achieved with either surgery or radiation for early-stage disease. Intraarterial administration has not improved the poor response to chemotherapy.

277. APPLYING BASIC CONCEPTS: INITIAL WORKUP: ANSWER: B
(*Isselbacher, 13/e, pp 1419-1420.*) Colonic diverticula result when the mucosa herniates through the muscularis at the point where the nutrient artery normally penetrates. This sac-like protrusion can become inflamed and involve the adjacent serosal surface when its lumen is filled with fecal debris and causes compromise of venous drainage from the diverticulum. Most cases present with left lower quadrant pain, fever, and leukocytosis and are managed with IV antibiotics. Non-inflamed diverticula may cause hematochezia when the adjacent nutrient artery is eroded by the fecal debris within the diverticular lumen. Often bleeding originates in right-sided colonic diverticula.

278. APPLYING BASIC CONCEPTS: INITIAL WORKUP: ANSWER: B
(Schwartz, 6/e, p 749.) Bronchial carcinoid tumors rarely produce the carcinoid syndrome. They are slow-growing, infrequently metastatic tumors that histologically resemble the carcinoid tumors of the small intestine. Over 80 percent arise in the major proximal bronchi and their intraluminal growth is responsible for the frequent presentation of bronchial obstruction. The only therapy for this lesion is operative resection since neither the primary tumor nor the infrequent lymph node metastasis is radiosensitive. The low malignant potential for this lesion is reflected by a long-term survival rate that approaches 90 percent.

279. HEALTH MAINTENANCE: INITIAL WORKUP: ANSWER: D
(Isselbacher, 13/e, chap 307. Jandl, chap 11.) The gene for glucose 6-phosphate dehydrogenase (G6PD) is located on the X chromosome; thus, G6PD deficiency is a sex-linked trait. Hemolytic anemia occurs much more commonly in males than in heterozygote female carriers, who usually are asymptomatic. Of the more than 100 variants of G6PD, the most commonly encountered variant of clinical significance in the United States is the A– type, which is found in about 15 percent of black males. It generally causes less severe hemolysis than the Mediterranean variant. Hemolysis usually is precipitated by an environmental oxidant stress, most commonly viral or bacterial infection. Certain drugs, such as antimalarial agents, sulfonamides, phenacetin, and vitamin K, also can trigger hemolysis. These oxidant stresses cause precipitation of hemoglobin, because affected persons are unable to maintain adequate intracellular levels of reduced glutathione. Precipitated hemoglobin forms Heinz bodies that are visualized only with supravital stains; these inclusions cause premature destruction of the red cells. The diagnosis should be considered in any person experiencing a hemolytic episode. However, since decreased G6PD levels are found mainly in older cells, a false negative test may be obtained during a hemolytic crisis, and the test should be repeated upon recovery.

280. HEALTH MAINTENANCE: CONTINUED CARE: ANSWER: B
(*Carr, pp 592-593, 602-605.*) Estrogen replacement therapy is useful in the prevention of osteoporosis and is felt to protect women against coronary heart disease. Postmenopausal estrogen users have decreased levels of low-density lipoprotein (LDL) and increased levels of high-density lipoprotein (HDL). Postmenopausal estrogen intake has not been shown to significantly increase the risk of ovarian cancer in women. Studies on its relation to breast cancer are more confusing, but at this time use of estrogen does not appear to increase the risk of breast cancer in postmenopausal women.

281. CLINICAL INTERVENTION: EMERGENCY: ANSWER: B
(Isselbacher, 13/e, chap 202.) The combination of hypotension and bradycardia suggests a vagal response in the setting of an acute myocardial infarction. Administration of the anticholinergic agent atropine is the treatment of choice. If the bradyarrhythmia and hypotension persist after 2.0 mg of atropine has been administered in divided doses, insertion of a temporary pacemaker is indicated. Isoproterenol should be avoided in patients with acute myocardial infarction since it may greatly increase myocardial oxygen consumption and thereby intensify ischemia. Volume replacement or inotropic support may be required if hypotension persists after correction of the bradyarrhythmia, but they are not indicated as initial therapies.

282. DIAGNOSTIC STUDIES: EMERGENCY: ANSWER: E
(*Isselbacher, 13/e, chap 114.*) Because a marked lymphocytosis characteristically is observed in children who have *Haemophilus pertussis* infection (whooping cough) and is rare in other respiratory illnesses, white blood cell count with differential would be useful in making the diagnosis. Blood cultures would be negative, and Gram stain of the sputum and chest and neck x-rays would show nonspecific changes. The diagnosis of pertussis is confirmed in most cases by nasopharyngeal culture.

283. CLINICAL THERAPEUTICS: CONTINUED CARE: ANSWER: A
(*Herbst, 2/e, pp 303-307.*) The marked effectiveness of the combined oral contraceptive pill, which contains a synthetic estrogen and a progestin, is related to its multiple antifertility actions. The primary effect is to suppress gonadotropins, thus inhibiting ovulation. The prolonged progestational effect also causes thickening of the cervical mucus and atrophic changes of the endometrium, thus impairing sperm penetrability and ovum implantation, respectively.

284. DIAGNOSIS: CONTINUED CARE: ANSWER: D
(Isselbacher, 13/e, chap 255.) The clinical history and x-ray presented in the question are consistent with toxic megacolon in association with severe ulcerative colitis. Toxic megacolon is most likely to occur when hypomotility agents, such as diphenoxylate or loperamide, are given to persons with severe colitis, or when such persons undergo a barium-enema radiographic procedure. In the case presented, a barium enema was not only dangerous but, in fact, unnecessary, because the presence of diarrhea and signs of systemic illness indicated that the disease no longer was limited to the rectum. Colonic perforation may also be associated with severe ulcerative colitis; the presence of subdiaphragmatic air on abdominal x-rays would be suggestive.

285. CLINICAL THERAPEUTICS: EMERGENCY: ANSWER: C
(Isselbacher, 13/e, chap 202.) The man described in the question probably has a right ventricular infarction complicating his inferior myocardial infarction, because right atrial pressure is elevated out of proportion to the left atrial (pulmonary capillary wedge) pressure. Cardiac output is probably depressed, given the low left-heart filling pressure. The best treatment consists of administration of fluids.

286. APPLYING BASIC CONCEPTS: EMERGENCY: ANSWER: B
(Cameron, 4/e, pp 785-791. Hardy, 2/e, pp 1002-1015.) Although the vast majority of pulmonary emboli are believed to originate in deep vein thrombosis of the legs (the remainder originating in the pelvic veins, right heart, and deep veins of the upper extremities), emboli in more than two-thirds of patients have clinically occult origins. A variety of diagnostic studies using impedance plethysmography, ^{125}I-fibrinogen scanning, contrast venography, radionuclide (blood pool) venography, ultrasonography, and computed tomography have been employed to identify the source of pulmonary emboli. While arteriovenous shunting in the lungs appears to play a role in the hypoxemia of pulmonary embolism, an increase in the ventilation-perfusion ratio of the affected areas, followed by reflex and, possibly, serotonin-mediated bronchoconstriction, is the main physiological derangement. An otherwise healthy patient who has less than 20 percent of the pulmonary vascular bed occluded would remain asymptomatic, and therefore the occlusion would not be discovered without screening studies.

287. DIAGNOSTIC STUDIES: INITIAL WORKUP: ANSWER: D
(Isselbacher, 13/e, chap 206.) The lateral-view chest film demonstrates calcification of the anterior pericardium, consistent with constrictive pericarditis. This pattern is seen in approximately one-half of patients with long-standing constriction, and pericardial thickening can often be confirmed by echocardiography. In patients with this disease, a pericardial knock is often heard 0.06 to 0.12 s after aortic valve closure, corresponding to the sudden cessation of ventricular filling. Murmurs are typically absent.

288. DIAGNOSIS: INITIAL WORKUP: ANSWER: A
(Isselbacher, 13/e, chap 290.) Behçet's syndrome, a recurrent disease of unknown cause, is characterized by painful oral and genital ulcers, eye inflammation, arthritis, central nervous system symptoms, thrombophlebitis, fever, and abdominal symptoms. The combination of fever, aphthous ulcers, arthritis, and abdominal pain may mimic inflammatory bowel disease, although central nervous system involvement (e.g., severe headache) and thrombophlebitis would make this diagnosis less likely. Whipple's disease is associated with arthritis, abdominal pain, and central nervous system disease, but not with aphthous ulcers and thrombophlebitis; also, Whipple's disease usually affects middle-aged men. Fever, arthritis, abdominal pain, and headache would be compatible with a diagnosis of systemic lupus erythematosus. However, the mucosal lesions of lupus are painless and occur on the hard and soft palate, and thrombophlebitis is not a characteristic feature.

289. PROGNOSIS: EMERGENCY: ANSWER: D
(Schwartz, 6/e, pp 1731-1732.) Testicular torsion occurs commonly in adolescents. The underlying pathology is secondary to an abnormally narrowed testicular mesentery with tunica vaginalis surrounding the testis and epididymis in a "bell-clapper" deformity. As the testis twists, it comes to lie in a higher position within the scrotum. Urinalysis is usually negative. Elevation will not provide a decrease in pain (negative Prehn's sign); a positive Prehn's sign might indicate epididymitis. A technetium-99m pertechnetate scan may be helpful in clarifying a confusing case; however, operation should not be delayed beyond 6 h from the time of onset of symptoms in order to maximize testicular salvage. This patient's presentation warrants immediate operation. The salvage rate for delay greater than 12 h is less than 20 percent. Both the affected and unaffected testes should undergo orchiopexy. Epididymitis usually occurs in sexually active males. Urinalysis is usually positive for inflammatory cells, and urethral discharge is often present.

290. DIAGNOSIS: INITIAL WORKUP: ANSWER: C
(Isselbacher, 13/e, chap 287.) Mixed connective tissue disease (MCTD) is a syndrome characterized by high titers of circulating antibodies to the ribonucleoprotein component of extractable nuclear antigen in association with clinical features similar to those of SLE, systemic sclerosis, polymyositis, and rheumatoid arthritis. The average patient with MCTD is a middle-aged woman with Raynaud's phenomenon who also has polyarthritis, sclerodactyly (including swollen hands), esophageal dysfunction, pulmonary fibrosis, and inflammatory myopathy. Cutaneous manifestations include telangiectasias on the face and hands, alopecia, a lupuslike heliotropic rash, and erythematous patches over the knuckles. Myopathy may involve severe weakness of proximal muscles associated with high levels of creatine phosphokinase and aldolase. Both pulmonary involvement and esophageal dysmotility are common, but frequently asymptomatic until quite advanced. Almost all patients have high titers of rheumatoid factor and antinuclear antibodies. Such antibodies are directed toward the ribonuclease-sensitive ribonucleoprotein component of the extractable nuclear antigen.

291. HEALTH MAINTENANCE: CONTINUED CARE: ANSWER: D
(*Barron, p 610.*) Patients at high risk for postpartum depression often have histories of depression or postpartum depression. They are more likely to be primiparous or older; they may have had a long interval between pregnancies or an unplanned pregnancy or be without a supportive partner. Prenatal intervention must include the obstetric team with family or peer support when possible. Postpartum depression is variable in duration, but occasionally will not resolve without hospitalization, therapy, or medication.

292. DIAGNOSIS: INITIAL WORKUP: ANSWER: E
(Isselbacher, 13/e, chap 299.) Pigmented villonodular synovitis, the cause of which is unknown, is a disorder of young adults that usually affects one joint only, frequently a knee. There is recurrent bleeding into the affected joint; the synovial fluid of that joint often contains blood and typically is dark brown in color, an indication of past bleeding from the synovium. The enlarged villi covering the synovium are made up of large numbers of round and polyhedral cells. Hemosiderin granules and cholesterol crystals can be identified in synovial cell cytoplasm as well as in interstitial spaces. Bone adjacent to the affected synovium can show evidence of erosion; however, invasion of other tissues does not occur. The synovial fluid findings in the case presented are incompatible with the diagnoses of atypical rheumatoid arthritis, incomplete Reiter's syndrome, and osteochondritis dissecans. Hemangioma usually presents in childhood.

293. PROGNOSIS: INITIAL WORKUP: ANSWER: C
(Schwartz, 6/e, pp 1731, 1764-1765.) Seminomas tend to grow slowly and metastasize late. They represent about 40 percent of malignant testicular tumors; embryonal cell carcinoma and teratocarcinoma each represents about 25 percent. Since most tumors have mixed elements, they are usually classified according to the most malignant cell type encountered, whatever the predominant cell type. When metastases occur, they are usually along the regional lymphatic drainage pathways to the iliac, aortic, and renal lymph nodes. Because of their slow growth and radiosensitivity, seminomas are associated with a 90 percent 5-year survival rate. Therapy generally consists of removing the affected testis and sampling the lymph nodes (usually external iliac) for evidence of metastasis. If metastases are present, radiation therapy is given locally to areas of known involvement. Radiation therapy is highly effective in seminoma, and metastatic disease may be palliated for extended periods.

294. CLINICAL INTERVENTION: INITIAL WORKUP: ANSWER: E
(*Isselbacher, 13/e, pp 1667-1668.*) Nonpurulent arthritis following an infection elsewhere in the body has been termed reactive arthritis. Reiter's syndrome is one such reactive arthritis most often associated with an enteric or urethral infection. The latter are especially common in males. As with many immunologic arthritides, there is a high association with the HLA-B27 antigen, 60 to 85 percent positivity in patients affected with reactive arthritis. Inflammation at the insertion site of tendons, enthesitis, occurs frequently in the ankles and feet. An asymmetric sacroiliitis can be a late sequela of Reiter's syndrome.

295. CLINICAL THERAPEUTICS: EMERGENCY: ANSWER: D
(Isselbacher, 13/e, chap 307. Byrne, Clin Haematol 15:413, 1986.) This young woman is suffering from a combination of hemolytic anemia with fragmented red cells in the absence of disseminated intravascular coagulation (DIC), thrombocytopenia, fever, mental status changes, and renal dysfunction, which is essentially pathognomonic of thrombotic thrombocytopenic purpura (TTP). The etiology of TTP is unknown, though immunologic and primary vasculopathic phenomena have been associated with this disorder. Pathologically, arteriolar hyalinization, which is also seen in DIC, may be noted. Seventy percent of patients with TTP improve with exchange transfusion or plasmapheresis. Glucocorticoids, antiplatelet agents, splenectomy, and vincristine have been of benefit to subsets of patients, but each is less effective and probably associated with a greater risk than therapeutic plasmapheresis.

296. PROGNOSIS: INITIAL WORKUP: ANSWER: A
(Isselbacher, 13/e, pp 1674-1675.) Wegener's granulomatosis is a rare disorder characterized by a granulomatous small vessel vasculitis with frequent involvement of the lungs, kidneys, and upper respiratory tract. Pulmonary lesions are often cavitary. Clinically, there may be hemoptysis, dyspnea, or chest pain. Renal involvement occurs in 75 percent of patients and can progress to renal failure if untreated. Treatment with cyclophosphamide will usually induce remission and thus renal failure is not inevitable. The presence of antineutrophil cytoplasmic antibody is a sensitive and specific marker for active Wegener's granulomatosis.

297. CLINICAL INTERVENTION: CONTINUED CARE: ANSWER: A
(Cameron, 4/e, pp 791-794.) The Greenfield filter pictured on the x-ray is used to interrupt migration of emboli to the lungs from the veins below the level of the filter. It is indicated in patients who sustain a recurrent pulmonary embolus despite adequate anticoagulant therapy or in patients with pulmonary emboli who cannot receive anticoagulants because of a contraindication (e.g, bleeding ulcer, intracranial hemorrhage). The filter is not used in patients who sustain a single pulmonary embolus. The filter is placed in the inferior vena cava just below the renal veins and therefore would not be effective for emboli that arise cephalad to its position.

298. DIAGNOSIS: INITIAL WORKUP: ANSWER: E
(Isselbacher, 13/e, chap 303. Henderson, 5/e, chap 24.) A slightly increased mean corpuscular volume and an inappropriately low reticulocyte count are characteristic of a macrocytic, hypoproliferative anemia. Iron-deficiency anemia is accompanied by microcytic red blood cell indices, and autoimmune hemolytic anemia typically is associated with reticulocytosis, unless a coexisting process, such as folate deficiency, interferes with the bone marrow erythropoietic response. Aplastic anemia and acute leukemia are unlikely diagnoses if white blood cell count and platelet count are normal. A macrocytic, hypoproliferative anemia in the older man described in the question would most likely be due to a myelodysplastic syndrome. A bone marrow examination with iron stain would be required to define the precise subtype of this heterogeneous disorder, which is characterized by a stem cell defect leading to disordered hematopoietic maturation. Given the normal platelet count and white blood cell count, either refractory anemia or refractory anemia with ringed sideroblasts is the most likely subtype. Certain acquired primary sideroblastic anemias, especially those without associated dysplastic changes in white cells or platelets, can be thought of as a defect in iron incorporation into heme and present with microcytosis.

299. APPLYING BASIC CONCEPTS: INITIAL WORKUP: ANSWER: B
(Youmans, 3/e, pp 3667-3676.) Peripheral nerve tumors include lesions of peripheral nerves, the adrenal gland nerve tissue, and the sympathetic chain. Schwannomas are peripheral nerve sheath tumors that arise from perineural fibroblasts (Schwann cells). Intracranial schwannomas most frequently originate in the vestibular branch of the eighth cranial nerve and represent 10 percent of all intracranial neoplasms. Symptoms include hearing loss, tinnitus, and vertigo. Malignant schwannomas are rare. Neurofibromas are also Schwann cell tumors but are histologically distinguishable from schwannomas. Neurofibromatosis (von Recklinghausen's disease) involves multiple peripheral nerve neoplasms. Neuronal tumors of peripheral nerves include ganglioneuroma, neuroblastoma, chemodectoma, and pheochromocytomas.

300. CLINICAL INTERVENTION: CONTINUED CARE: ANSWER: E
(*Herbst, 2/e, p 349.*) Vasectomy is performed by isolating the vas deferens, cutting it, and closing the ends by either fulguration or ligation. Complications that may arise include hematoma in up to 5 percent of subjects, sperm granulomas (inflammatory responses to sperm leakage), spontaneous reanastomosis, and, rarely, infections.

301. CLINICAL INTERVENTION: INITIAL WORKUP: ANSWER: C
(Youmans, 3/e, pp 2970-2972, 3223-3238.) Craniopharyngiomas are cystic tumors with areas of calcification and originate in the epithelial remnants of Rathke's pouch. These usually benign tumors are found in the sellar and suprasellar region and lead to compression of the pituitary, optic tracts, and third ventricle. As a result they can present with symptoms of visual disturbance, endocrine dysfunction, headache, or even hydrocephalus. Craniopharyngiomas are most commonly found in children but may also present in adulthood. Treatment consists of subfrontal or transsphenoidal excision with adjuvant radiotherapy if total removal is not possible.

302. DIAGNOSTIC STUDIES: INITIAL WORKUP: ANSWER: C
(Isselbacher, 13/e, chaps 57, 315.) A marked prolongation of the prothrombin time with a normal partial thromboplastin time localizes the hemostatic defect to the extrinsic limb of the coagulation cascade. Congenital factor VII deficiency is a rare, autosomal recessive disorder. Factor VIII deficiency and the presence of specific inhibitors directed towards a coagulation factor (most commonly factor VIII) would be associated with a prolongation of the partial thromboplastin time. Nonspecific inhibitors (lupus anticoagulants) most commonly are associated with prolongation of the partial thromboplastin time and occasionally with prolongation of the prothrombin time (particularly when hypoprothrombinemia is present). Patients with alpha$_2$-antiplasmin deficiency have a bleeding disorder associated with accelerated clot lysis. Both the prothrombin time and the partial thromboplastin time are normal in these persons.

303. PROGNOSIS: INITIAL WORKUP: ANSWER: E
(Isselbacher, 13/e, chap 304.) Antiparietal-cell antibodies are detected in 90 percent of persons with pernicious anemia but also in persons with atrophic gastritis and 10 to 15 percent of an unselected patient population. Although folate in large doses can correct the megaloblastic anemia of pernicious anemia, it does not correct the neurologic abnormalities. Megaloblastic anemias are characterized by ineffective erythropoiesis and bone marrow erythroid hyperplasia. Hypergastrinemia accompanies the achlorhydria of pernicious anemia. Marrow morphology begins to improve within hours of parenteral B_{12} therapy; reticulocytosis peaks in 1 week. Life-threatening hypokalemia may occur early in the course of therapy.

304. CLINICAL THERAPEUTICS: CONTINUED CARE: ANSWER: A
(Behrman, 3/e, chap 18.) An inadequate corpus luteal phase may explain repeated abortion in early pregnancy. Natural progesterone may be useful in supplying additional progesterone until the placenta is functioning sufficiently. Serum progesterone concentrations two standard deviations below that anticipated during the luteal phase is evidence of an inadequate corpus luteum. Progesterone therapy requires 25-mg vaginal suppositories twice daily within 2 days of the thermogenic rise in basal body temperature. The medicine is continued for 6 weeks or until menstrual bleeding occurs. Intramuscular injection of progesterone in oil, 12.5 mg daily, may be used instead, but synthetic progestins are discouraged because of potential teratogenic effects.

305. CLINICAL INTERVENTION: CONTINUED CARE: ANSWER: D
(*Isselbacher, 13/e, chap 59. Malech, N Engl J Med 317:687, 1987.*) This child most likely has chronic granulomatous disease (CGD), a group of inherited disorders that have in common defective oxidative metabolism of neutrophils. This defect results in a heightened susceptibility to infection with catalase-positive organisms such as staphylococci and *Aspergillus*. The diagnosis can be made by demonstrating abnormal neutrophil reduction of nitroblue tetrazolium. Recent studies have suggested that interferon-gamma may be useful in correcting the neutrophil dysfunction characteristic of CGD. Most patients with isolated deficiency of myeloperoxidase are not at increased risk for infection unless another defect is present, in which case infection with *Candida albicans* may be a problem. Decreased serum levels of immunoglobulins predispose to infection with encapsulated organisms such as *Haemophilus* and streptococci, while defects in T-lymphocyte function are manifested as infection with viruses and protozoal pathogens such as *Pneumocystis carinii*.

306. HEALTH MAINTENANCE: CONTINUED CARE: ANSWER: E
(*Creasy, 2/e, pp 1167-1169.*) Maternal diabetes, especially of the milder classes, is associated with macrosomia in the fetus. Glucose crosses the placenta freely by facilitated diffusion, but insulin does not. The fetus, in response to the chronic glucose load, secretes increased quantities of insulin. Insulin acts as a growth hormone in the fetus, and the fetus becomes macrosomic. At delivery, the fetus is removed from the relatively glucose-rich maternal environment but continues to secrete increased amounts of insulin. Thus, the fetus may become hypoglycemic in the early hours of life unless early feedings, sometimes even intravenous glucose, are begun. Hypocalcemia may occur in as many as one-fourth of infants of diabetic mothers, possibly as a result of fetal parathyroid suppression stemming from maternal hypercalcemia. Lastly, fetal lung maturity, as measured by the lecithin-to-sphingomyelin ratio, may be delayed, especially in the infants of mothers who have mild diabetes.

307. HEALTH MAINTENANCE: INITIAL WORKUP: ANSWER: A
(*Isselbacher, 13/e, chap 161.*) The physical signs and symptoms listed in the question suggest infection with *Candida albicans*. *C. albicans* infections occur in several clinical settings: diabetes in poor control; broad-spectrum antibiotic therapy; chronic mucocutaneous candidiasis syndrome; and others. Although some of these conditions may be associated with elevated serum levels of immunoglobulins A and E, these are nonspecific findings. On the other hand, a significantly elevated blood glucose concentration would make the diagnosis of diabetes almost certain. In complement deficiency or uremia, the defects in host defense are not characteristically manifested by vaginal candidiasis.

308. DIAGNOSTIC STUDIES: CONTINUED CARE: ANSWER: A
(*Isselbacher, 13/e, chap 179.*) Cryptosporidia, which are protozoa, cannot be cultured from the stool. They stain with iodine but not Gram stain. Investigational serologic tests appear promising but are not readily available. Because of their small size (5 mm) and lack of motility, detection of cysts by wet mounts is very difficult. By using acid-fast stains or rhodamine fluorescence, even a few cysts can be detected easily and the diagnosis of cryptosporidiosis made.

309. APPLYING BASIC CONCEPTS: INITIAL WORKUP: ANSWER: C
(Youmans, 3/e, pp 2664-2694.) The intervertebral disk is susceptible to degenerative changes especially in the lower cervical and lower lumbar spine. This can lead to a thinning of the annulus fibrosis and loss of its fibrocartilage. Marked mechanical stresses are another means of damage when they cause tears in the annulus. Herniation of a portion of the nucleus pulposus can result from either problem. Not all such herniations are symptomatic, but those in the lumbar region most often lead to numbness or pain or both. Ninety-five percent of lumbar herniations are at L4-L5 or L5-S1. A posterolateral herniation in the lumbar region impinges on the anterior and posterior nerve roots of the inferior intervertebral foramen. Thus, a herniation at the L4-L5 interspace will compress the fifth lumbar roots. The anterior roots of L5 serves the anterior crural and peroneal muscles. The most common sequela of compression is weakness of dorsiflexion of the great toe. The L5 posterior root serves the dermatome from the anterolateral aspect of the leg to the dorsum and the medial aspect of the foot. Compression here can result in pain on the dorsum of the foot. Weakness on plantar flexion and sensory deficit on the lateral aspect of the foot are symptoms associated with compression of the first sacral roots common with posterolateral herniations at L5-S1.

310. HISTORY AND PHYSICAL: EMERGENCY: ANSWER: D
(*Isselbacher, 13/e, chap 113.*) Legionnaire's disease is caused by *Legionella pneumophila*. It occurs sporadically or in outbreaks and often begins with myalgias, headache, and fever. Diarrhea and delirium also are early features in many cases. Gastrointestinal symptoms should suggest the possibility of this diagnosis, particularly in persons who have severe pneumonia, scant production of sputum, and other extrapulmonary abnormalities. Of the other organisms listed in the question, all can cause pneumonia; *Mycoplasma pneumoniae* infection is most likely to be confused with Legionnaire's disease.

311. APPLYING BASIC CONCEPTS: INITIAL WORKUP: ANSWER: C
(Schwartz, 6/e, pp 650-655.) These round tumors have a rubbery consistency and are slow-growing; all are potentially malignant. Unless adequately excised, they tend to recur locally in a high percentage of cases. The sites most commonly affected by pleomorphic adenomas of the salivary glands are the lips, tongue, and palate.

312. APPLYING BASIC CONCEPTS: INITIAL WORKUP: ANSWER: D
(*Isselbacher, 13/e, chap 105.*) *Listeria monocytogenes* is a gram-positive motile bacillus that tends to infect infants as well as persons over the age of 55 years. Major illnesses in both groups are meningitis and other forms of central nervous system infection. Many of the older patients are immunosuppressed because of disease (e.g., cancer), immunosuppressive drug therapy, or both. Endocarditis, peritonitis, hepatitis, and conjunctivitis also can be caused by *Listeria* infection.

313. DIAGNOSIS: CONTINUED CARE: ANSWER: A
(Behrman, 14/e, pp 948-958.) The finding of hydramnios signals high intestinal obstruction, signs of which include abdominal distention and early and repeated regurgitation. Distention may not be present if the obstruction is very high or if vomiting keeps the intestine decompressed. The bile-stained vomitus of the infant places the obstruction distal to the ampulla of Vater, eliminating esophageal atresia and pyloric stenosis from consideration. The "double bubble" sign on the x-ray is characteristic of duodenal atresia, which is compatible with the history. Midgut volvulus, which may obstruct the bowel in the area of the duodenojejunal junction, most often produces signs after an affected infant is 3 or 4 days old, and several loops of small bowel are typically seen on x-ray. Gastric duplication does not usually produce intestinal obstruction; a cystic mass may be palpated on abdominal examination.

314. DIAGNOSIS: INITIAL WORKUP: ANSWER: A
(*Isselbacher, 13/e, chap 130.*) The diagnosis of a tuberculous pleural effusion is suggested by the following set of pleural-fluid findings: color, clear yellow; pH, < 7.20; protein, > 30 g/L; glucose, < 1.2 mmol/L (25 mg/dL); lactate dehydrogenase (LDH), > 450 U/mL; and a lymphocytosis. Tubercle bacilli rarely are identified on a smear of infected pleural fluid, and cultures are positive in no more than one-quarter of cases. Antituberculous treatment should commence as soon as the diagnosis is suspected.

315. DIAGNOSIS: EMERGENCY: ANSWER: A
(*Isselbacher, 13/e, chap 89.*) The findings on pelvic examination coupled with the elevated sedimentation rate in this setting strongly suggest acute pelvic inflammatory disease (PID). About 5 percent of women with PID will have associated perihepatitis, termed the Fitz-Hugh-Curtis syndrome, manifested by pleuritic pain of the right upper quadrant and tenderness on palpation, along with normal liver function tests and ultrasound of the right upper quadrant. Although for many years *N. gonorrhoeae* was considered to be the primary pathogen in this condition, chlamydial salpingitis is now the most common associated finding.

316. CLINICAL THERAPEUTICS: EMERGENCY: ANSWER: C
(*Isselbacher, 13/e, chap 89.*) It is important to pick a well-tolerated regimen with good activity against both *N. gonorrhoeae* (including penicillinase-producing strains) and *C. trachomatis* for the treatment of patients with severe pelvic inflammatory disease. Activity against vaginal anaerobes and members of the Enterobacteriaceae family, which may also play a role in the pathogenesis of this disorder, would also be desirable. A combination of doxycycline and cefoxitin offers the broad-spectrum coverage required for optimal treatment. Clindamycin plus gentamicin acutely, plus a 2-week course of doxycycline to definitively treat *C. trachomatis*, is an acceptable alternative regimen. The combination of metronidazole and gentamicin lacks adequate coverage against both *Chlamydia* and *N. gonorrhoeae* and is therefore not appropriate in this setting.

317. CLINICAL INTERVENTION: EMERGENCY: ANSWER: C
(Hall, p 2053.) The immediate treatment in the emergency room is to remove any remaining alkaline material from the eye to minimize the chemical injury. While the other choices may be performed in the emergency room, the first maneuver is to irrigate the alkaline away.

318. CLINICAL INTERVENTION: EMERGENCY: ANSWER: D

(Isselbacher, 13/e, p 2348.) While all of the other choices may be urgent problems, a central retinal artery occlusion is an emergency in which moments count. Retinal tissue can become irreversibly damaged with 20 or 30 minutes of ischemia. Immediate initiation of treatment for central retinal artery occlusion may limit the extent of ischemia. The goal is to cause the clot to move distally in the circulation and limit the central retinal artery occlusion to a branch retinal artery occlusion, minimizing the affected area of retina.

319. APPLYING BASIC CONCEPTS: INITIAL WORKUP: ANSWER: B

(Schwartz, 6/e, pp 963-964.) Atherosclerotic occlusion of the subclavian artery proximal to the vertebral artery is the anatomical situation that results in the subclavian steal syndrome. On being subjected to exercise the involved extremity (usually left) develops relative ischemia, which gives rise to reversal of flow through the vertebral artery with consequent diminished flow to the brain. The upper extremity symptom is intermittent claudication. Venous occlusive disease is not a feature of the syndrome. The operative procedure for treating the subclavian steal syndrome consists of delivering blood to the extremity by creating either a carotid-subclavian or axillo-axillary bypass.

320. PROGNOSIS: CONTINUED CARE: ANSWER: E

(*Berek, p 66.*) The extent (or stage) and the volume of a tumor are probably the most important prognostic considerations in the management of women who have ovarian epithelial carcinoma. However, on a stage-for-stage basis, women who have well-differentiated tumors have better prognoses than women who have poorly differentiated tumors. The presence of ascites or peritoneal washings that are cytologically positive for malignant cells decreases the 5-year survival of affected women.

321. DIAGNOSTIC STUDIES: CONTINUED CARE: ANSWER: A

(Isselbacher, 13/e, chap 192.) A gradient between the left atrium (as measured by the pulmonary capillary wedge tracing) and the left ventricle in diastole indicates mitral stenosis as exemplified by the woman with a history of rheumatic fever and hemoptysis. The intravenous drug abuser with mitral regurgitation caused by a mitral valve vegetation would exhibit large *v* waves on the pulmonary capillary wedge tracing. The aortic regurgitation associated with Marfan's syndrome would cause an equilibration between left ventricular and peripheral pressures. A feature of severe aortic regurgitation occurs when left ventricular pressure exceeds pulmonary capillary wedge (i.e., left atrial) pressure during early diastole, which results in premature mitral valve closure. In aortic stenosis, as exemplified by the elderly man with left ventricular hypertrophy, the left ventricular pressure is higher than aortic pressure during systole. In pericardial tamponade, as might be seen in the patient with lymphoma, there is equalization of right and left diastolic pressures.

322. DIAGNOSIS: CONTINUED CARE: ANSWERS: A, D

(*Cunningham, 18/e, p 577. Jones, 4/e, pp 572-573.*) An infant with Potter syndrome generally has a breech presentation. After birth, the baby is never able to ventilate adequately. These infants rarely survive more than a few hours. The primary lesion in Potter syndrome is thought to be renal. Because of renal agenesis, urine output is impossible, and oligohydramnios results. Oligohydramnios is believed to lead to pulmonary hypoplasia, because lack of amniotic fluid somehow restricts normal lung development. The characteristic facial anomalies (large, low-set ears and flattened nose) are thought to be related to pressure on the face increased by a lack of cushioning amniotic fluid. The diagnosis of Potter syndrome has been made antenatally with the aid of ultrasonography. Demonstration of a fetal bladder that fills and empties should rule out Potter syndrome. The absence of evidence of a bladder, despite repeated ultrasonographic examinations, would be compatible with the diagnosis. Amnion nodosum, another common finding in Potter syndrome, consists of multiple opaque nodules in the amnion. Their cause is not clear, but they represent fetal squames that have become "parasitic" on the membranes.

323. DIAGNOSIS: CONTINUED CARE: ANSWERS: B, E

(*Charles, p 340. Evans, pp 111-112. Remington, 3/e, p 5.*) Rubella syndrome in the newborn secondary to rubella infection during pregnancy (especially, not exclusively, during the first trimester) is well known. Although cytomegalovirus infection is less familiar, it is thought to cause congenital anomalies in about 500 newborns every year in the United States. The abnormalities are usually in the central nervous system and include microcephaly, cerebral calcifications, deafness, and other mental and motor disabilities. Although there have been some suggestions that influenza epidemics have led to a subsequent rise in the incidence of childhood leukemia, this relationship has not been established; in fact, there is no proof that influenza is associated with any anomalies. Mumps is relatively common during pregnancy, but prospective studies have failed to show any associated congenital anomalies.

324. CLINICAL INTERVENTION: CONTINUED CARE: ANSWERS: B, C, E

(*Eden, pp 809-822.*) In general, the presence of fetal movements is a reassuring sign of fetal health. However, the absence of fetal activity requires further assessment before one can conclude that fetal compromise exists. The contraction stress test (CST) requires uterine contractions of moderate intensity lasting 40 to 60 s with a frequency of 3 in 10 min. The basis for this test is the response to uterine contractions of the fetus at risk for uteroplacental insufficiency. A reactive nonstress test (NST) requires at least 2 accelerations of the fetal heart rate of 15 beats per minute and 15 s duration during a 20-min period. The biophysical profile (BPP) adds to the NST the use of real-time ultrasound to assess fetal breathing movement, gross body movement, fetal tone, and amniotic fluid volume. There is a great deal of controversy over which test is best. Recent studies have shown that both NST and BPP are valuable predictors of normal outcome. Overall, the BPP and CST appear to be associated with the lowest incidence of intrauterine death.

325. HISTORY AND PHYSICAL: INITIAL WORKUP: ANSWER: C

(Isselbacher, 13/e, chap 247.) Older men are the most frequent victims of carcinoma of the bladder. Transitional cell carcinoma, the most common histologic subtype of cancer of the bladder in this country, is associated with a more favorable prognosis than is adenocarcinoma or squamous carcinoma. Squamous carcinomas are more frequent in Egypt, where the prevalence of *Schistosoma haematobium* is high. The prognosis in cancer of the bladder is highly linked to the stage of the disease at presentation: muscular or perivascular fat invasion offers a much bleaker outlook (45 percent 5-year survival) than

does disease confined to the mucosa. Risk factors for cancer of the bladder include exposure to the aromatic amines (cigarette smoke and products of the dye, rubber, and chemical industries), but not positive family history, as in the case of renal carcinoma. Chronic bladder irritation, such as that produced by the metabolites of cyclophosphamide as well as by recurrent stones or infections, also leads to a higher incidence of carcinoma of the bladder.

326. DIAGNOSTIC STUDIES: CONTINUED CARE: ANSWER: C
(Isselbacher, 13/e, chap 365.) CT scanning still remains the procedure of choice in the acute setting when rapid information about a suddenly deteriorating patient is required. It has a high specificity for demonstrating acute hemorrhage, and in that respect is superior to MRI. Calcifications within the brain and bony lesions are also better delineated on CT than on MRI. However, MRI has added diagnostic potential in a number of circumstances, including screening for metastatic disease (particularly if gadolinium enhancement is used), imaging demyelinating diseases, and identifying the presence of aneurysms and arteriovenous malformations as well as developmental malformations, posterior fossa lesions, and almost all spinal cord lesions—including vertebral osteomyelitis, epidural abscess, herniated disks, and syringomyelia.

327. CLINICAL THERAPEUTICS: CONTINUED CARE: ANSWER: E
(Isselbacher, 13/e, chap 195.) Elderly persons are particularly prone to develop digitalis intoxication at relatively low doses and apparently normal serum levels (< 2.0 pg/L). Exacerbating factors in the development of toxicity are hypoxemia and hypercalcemia. Potassium wasting and, perhaps, hypomagnesemia from potent loop diuretics also can foster toxicity. By mechanisms not yet elucidated, quinidine can increase the serum levels of digoxin, thereby inducing toxicity. Hyperthyroidism tends to decrease the efficacy of digitalis, while hypothyroidism enhances the likelihood of toxicity.

328. HEALTH MAINTENANCE: CONTINUED CARE: ANSWER: C
(Isselbacher, 13/e, chap 257. Vogelstein, N Engl J Med 319:595, 1988.) The specific cause of colon cancer is unknown, although recent studies reveal an excess of genetic allele loss in advanced colonic neoplasia. However, certain diseases are known to increase the risk of development of cancer of the colon. Crohn's colitis is associated with an increased risk of colon cancer, although the risk is less than that for patients with ulcerative colitis. Colon cancer has been observed to occur with increased frequency in patients with uterine cancer. Patients with adenomatous polyps are at higher risk for the subsequent development of colon cancer than is the general population. Therefore, such patients should have periodic follow-up examinations. Despite the importance of these risk factors, only 1 percent of persons with colon cancer have an identifiable risk factor other than age. The polyps in juvenile polyposis are hamartomatous and have no malignant potential. Colonic neoplasms at a site distal to the ureteral implant have been noted to occur 15 to 30 years after uterosigmoidostomy.

329. DIAGNOSTIC STUDIES: INITIAL WORKUP: ANSWER: D
(*Isselbacher, 13/e, p 1487.*) In this setting the finding of an elevated AMA is suggestive of PBC but would require confirmation with liver biopsy. Hyperlipidemia is a usual feature and can be manifested by xanthelasmas and xanthomas. Copper levels are generally high in cholestatic states including PBC. Due to the bile salt deficiency associated with PBC, there is insufficient fat-soluble vitamin resorption and prolongation of the prothrombin time. Sicca syndrome occurs in 75 percent of patients with PBC.

330. PROGNOSIS: CONTINUED CARE: ANSWER: A
(*Droegemueller, pp 834-835.*) Ovarian carcinoma, though the third most common malignancy of gynecologic origin (after endometrial and cervical cancer), is associated with the highest mortality among the common gynecologic malignancies. The inability of routine screening tests to diagnose this malignancy in an early stage, in contrast to the efficacy of the Pap smear in detecting cervical cancer, is chiefly responsible for the high mortality. Most patients have advanced disease by the time their symptoms appear. Environmental, cultural, socioeconomic, and dietary factors all may play a role in the development of ovarian cancer.

331. CLINICAL INTERVENTION: CONTINUED CARE: ANSWER: B
(Isselbacher, 13/e, chap 254.) The histologic specimen pictured in the question shows villous atrophy, crypt hyperplasia, and inflammation typical of intestinal changes in nontropical sprue (celiac disease), an illness with a high incidence in Ireland. The disease is associated with an increased incidence of histocompatibility antigens HLA-B8 and HLA-DW3. Although two-thirds of symptomatic cases present in childhood, the onset of clinical symptoms of malabsorption may occur at any age. Persons with subclinical sprue during adolescence may have mild growth retardation and may be smaller than their siblings. Because the villous absorptive surface is markedly reduced in affected persons, an acquired lactase deficiency is often present and causes symptoms of milk intolerance. A strict gluten-free diet or use of corticosteroids usually relieves symptoms and signs of malabsorption and promotes restoration of normal jejunal histology. A malabsorptive syndrome associated with abdominal pain, arthralgias, low-grade fever, and lymphadenopathy is not typical of celiac disease and should suggest another diagnosis, such as Whipple's disease or lymphoma.

332. HEALTH MAINTENANCE: CONTINUED CARE: ANSWER: E
(Isselbacher, 13/e, chap 317.) The value of screening mammography in reducing the mortality rate in breast cancer in those over age 40 is well-established. Current guidelines dictate a baseline mammogram between ages 35 and 40, every other year from ages 40 to 49, and annually thereafter. Mammograms should be supplemented by an annual professional breast examination and monthly breast self-examinations. Pelvic examinations and Pap smears should be done annually until three consecutive normal studies are obtained, whereupon the frequency may be reduced. To reduce the incidence of colorectal neoplasia, annual digital rectal examinations and testing for occult blood in the stool are indicated. Though sigmoidoscopic examinations are suggested every 3 to 5 years after two initial negative tests 1 year apart, colonoscopy is not presently recommended as a routine screening procedure.

333. HISTORY AND PHYSICAL: INITIAL WORKUP: ANSWER: B
(Isselbacher, 13/e, chap 188.) Inspiration, which augments systemic venous return because of negative intrathoracic pressure, will cause accentuation of right-sided murmurs. Prolonged expiratory pressure against a closed glottis (Valsalva maneuver) reduces the intensity of most murmurs by diminishing both right and left ventricular filling. By reducing filling, and thereby reducing chamber size, the murmurs of hypertrophic cardiomyopathy and mitral valve prolapse will increase. The cycle following a premature ventricular beat will have a larger stroke volume so the gradient across an obstructed semilunar valve (aortic or pulmonary) will increase, thereby leading to a louder murmur. Squatting, which increases both venous return and chamber size as well as systemic arterial resistance, increases most murmurs except those due to hypertrophic cardiomyopathy and mitral valve prolapse. Sustained handgrip, which increases heart rate and systemic arterial pressure, often accentuates the murmurs of mitral stenosis and mitral regurgitation by impeding outflow and by decreasing diastolic filling.

334. DIAGNOSIS: INITIAL WORKUP: ANSWER: B

(Isselbacher, 13/e, chap 339.) The clinical situation described in the question is characteristic of congenital adrenal hyperplasia due to deficiency of either C-21 hydroxylase or 3 β-ol-dehydrogenase. Urinary 17-ketosteroids are elevated in both disorders, whereas urinary pregnanediol and pregnanetriol and plasma 17-hydroxyprogesterone and androstenedione levels are elevated in association with C-21 hydroxylase deficiency. Plasma 11-deoxycortisol is elevated in C-11 hydroxylase deficiency, a disorder producing hypertension owing to overproduction of mineralocorticoids and consequently not associated with vomiting and volume depletion.

335. CLINICAL INTERVENTION: EMERGENCY: ANSWER: C

(Isselbacher, 13/e, chap 210.) Complications of dissection of the aorta include loss of a major pulse, dissection into the pericardial or pleural space, and acute aortic regurgitation. When these events occur, surgical intervention is required. Because the risk of these complications is higher in persons with dissection of the ascending aorta, these persons usually are treated surgically. In contrast, persons with dissection of the descending aorta often can be treated medically. Persistence of pain, which suggests that dissection is continuing, is another indication for surgery.

336. HISTORY AND PHYSICAL: INITIAL WORKUP: ANSWER: E

(Isselbacher, 13/e, chap 200.) Two major criteria or one major and two minor criteria indicate a high probability of rheumatic fever in the presence of evidence of preceding streptococcal infection (history of scarlet fever, elevated ASO titer, or positive throat culture). The major criteria include carditis (new heart murmur, increase in heart size, pericardial friction rub, or CHF), polyarthritis, chorea (usually a delayed manifestation), erythema marginatum, and subcutaneous nodules. The minor criteria, which are relatively common and nonspecific, include fever, arthralgia, previous rheumatic fever or rheumatic heart disease, elevated erythrocyte sedimentation rate (ESR), or prolonged PR interval.

337. CLINICAL THERAPEUTICS: EMERGENCY: ANSWER: E

(*Isselbacher, 13/e, pp 1133-1134.*) Classification of aortic dissections depends on the involvement of the ascending aorta. With ascending aortic involvement, the dissection is classified as Debakey type I, and with coexistent extension into the descending aorta, Debakey type II. Debakey type III dissections involve the descending aorta only. The Stanford classification groups the DeBakey types I and II into type A, and Debakey type III is equivalent to Stanford type B. Involvement of the ascending aorta is an indication for surgical treatment but temporizing treatment with beta-blockers and nitroprusside is indicated in aortic dissection unless there is concomitant hypotension. The in-hospital mortality is similar for surgically and medically treated patients with acute aortic dissection; however, it is important to understand that the patient groups are different. Surgically treated patients will have ascending aortic involvement and may have significant complications from the dissection, such as hemopericardium, aortic regurgitation, myocardial infarction, renal or superior mesenteric artery involvement, etc. Patients with medically treated dissections by definition do not have these complications or involvement of the ascending aorta. Predisposing conditions for the development of aortic aneurysms include bicuspid aortic valve, coarctation, hypertension (occuring in 70 percent of such patients), and cystic medial necrosis, as well as other connective tissue abnormalities. Presenting symptoms include tearing chest pain with sudden onset, diaphoresis, and dyspnea. Additional symptoms relate to involvement of major arterial branches, i.e., coronary, carotid, renal. Widening of the mediastinum and pleural effusion, usually left-sided, are common chest x-ray findings.

338. CLINICAL INTERVENTION: CONTINUED CARE: ANSWER: A
(*Evans, pp 238-239.*) Amniocentesis, cordocentesis, and chorionic villus sampling are techniques of obtaining fetal tissues that are amenable to cytogenetic analysis. Amniotic fluid cells require tissue culture to obtain adequate cell numbers for analysis. Chorionic villi can be harvested "directly" for extremely rapid diagnosis or can be cultured for higher banding (increased detail). Fetal blood obtained by cordocentesis (or percutaneous umbilical blood sampling [PUBS]) requires 2 to 3 days' culturing before a karyotype is obtained.

339. CLINICAL INTERVENTION: CONTINUED CARE: ANSWER: E
(Isselbacher, 13/e, chap 203.) Any patient with recent onset of severe and frequent angina, accelerating angina, or angina at rest is considered to have unstable angina. Such patients are likely to have one or more stenoses in major coronary arteries and require emergent management. Hospitalization with identification and treatment of predisposing conditions (heart failure, fever, thyrotoxicosis) is indicated. Since thrombus formation frequently complicates this condition, intravenous heparin followed by oral aspirin should be given. Beta blockers and calcium channel blocking drugs should be administered if possible. Antiarrhythmics are only required in the presence of specific arrhythmias. Intravenous nitroglycerin is effective, but requires continuous blood pressure monitoring.

340. HEALTH MAINTENANCE: CONTINUED CARE: ANSWER: B
(Isselbacher, 13/e, chap 211.) Conditions associated with stasis, vascular damage, or hypercoagulability lead to an increased risk for deep venous thrombosis. Risk is increased by any condition leading to immobility, such as recuperation after a myocardial infarction (of any severity), a major thoracic resection (even if the cancer was completely resected), and trauma or operation involving the hip or leg. A wrist fracture in an elderly woman would probably not lead to any increased risk if her baseline mobility was present. Hypercoagulable states include systemic cancers; pregnancy; exogenous or endogenous estrogens; deficiencies of antithrombin III, protein C, and protein S; circulating lupus anticoagulant (manifested by elevated partial thromboplastin time); or myeloproliferative disease.

341. HEALTH MAINTENANCE: CONTINUED CARE: ANSWER: C
(Isselbacher, 13/e, chap 279. Curran, Science 239:610, 1988.) Among the U.S. cases of AIDS in adults, 60 percent are in homosexual men who do not use intravenous drugs; however, attack rates have precipitously declined in the homosexual community, probably owing to behavior modification. On the other hand, infections continue to rise among intravenous drug users. Because of blood donor screening and heat treatment of factor VIII concentrates, the rate of seroconversion in hemophiliacs is dropping. Blood donor screening reduces the risk of exposure to HIV in a single unit of blood to between 1/40,000 and 1/250,000. Pediatric AIDS arises mainly in infants born to mothers who are intravenous drug users or sexual partners of intravenous drug users. The remainder of pediatric AIDS patients are hemophiliacs or recipients of blood transfusions. The overall prevalence of HIV infection is quite low: about 0.04 percent of blood donors, who are a low-risk group because of the voluntary exclusion of high-risk individuals, to 0.15 percent of U.S. military recruits, a group relatively high in risk because of sexual activity and socioeconomic status. There is a small but real risk of seroconversion in those who are exposed to HIV-contaminated materials at the work place; less than 0.5 percent of those who have sustained penetrating injuries or whose mucosae have been splashed with blood from AIDS patients have become infected.

342. HEALTH MAINTENANCE: CONTINUED CARE: ANSWER: C
(*Mandell, 3/e, pp 2092-2100. Remington, 3/e, pp 89-95.*) Toxoplasmosis, a protozoal infection caused by *Toxoplasma gondii,* can result from ingestion of raw or undercooked meat infected by the organism or from contact with infected cat feces. Its incidence in pregnant women is estimated to be 1 in every 150 to 700 pregnancies. Infection early in pregnancy may cause abortion; later in pregnancy, however, the fetus may become infected. A small number of infected infants develop involvement of the central nervous system or the eye; most infants who have the disease, however, escape serious clinical problems.

343. DIAGNOSIS: INITIAL WORKUP: ANSWER: B
(Isselbacher, 13/e, chap 279.) AIDS is characterized by the infection of T4+ lymphocytes by the AIDS retrovirus (HTLV-III/LAV), with subsequent deficiency in numbers and functions of this T-cell subpopulation, which includes the important helper-inducer cells necessary for production of a variety of immune responses. Thus, there is a defect in the response of T cells to soluble antigen and to mitogenic substances such as phytohemagglutinin and concanavalin A. Natural killer cell function is abnormal and may be augmented in vitro by addition of the lymphokine interleukin 2. There is polyclonal activation of B lymphocytes, with a resultant increase in serum immunoglobulin levels and occasional production of autoantibodies.

344. CLINICAL INTERVENTION: EMERGENCY: ANSWER: D
(Isselbacher, 13/e, chap 279.) The clinical situation suggests the diagnosis of the acquired immunodeficiency syndrome (AIDS). *M. pneumoniae*, while a frequent cause of mild community-acquired pneumonia in the otherwise normal host, is not commonly associated with AIDS. *P. carinii*, a protozoal pathogen, is the most frequent cause of respiratory disease in the AIDS patient; it affects approximately 60 percent of such patients some time during the course of their illness. Both cytomegalovirus and *C. neoformans* are less common but significant respiratory pathogens in this patient population. Tuberculosis must always be considered in an AIDS patient with pulmonary symptoms. Tuberculous dissemination occurs frequently.

345. HISTORY AND PHYSICAL: CONTINUED CARE: ANSWER: C
(Isselbacher, 13/e, chap 255.) Peripheral arthritis and spondyloarthropathy can be associated with inflammatory bowel disease. The characteristic peripheral arthritis, which is more commonly associated with colonic disease than with small-bowel involvement alone, involves a few joints in the lower extremities, usually in an asymmetrical fashion, and resolves in a few months without residual joint damage. The presence and activity of peripheral arthritis are related to the extent and activity of colonic involvement. In contrast, the presence and activity of spondylitis are not related to the activity of bowel disease. This form of spondyloarthropathy behaves very much like ankylosing spondylitis and may even precede the emergence of bowel disease by many years.

346. HEALTH MAINTENANCE: CONTINUED CARE: ANSWER: C
(*Isselbacher, 13/e, chap 179.*) The infective cysts of *G. lamblia* can survive for several months in cold water and have been responsible for large epidemics in communities such as Vail, Colorado. Immunity to *Giardia* is not well understood, but there is no increased incidence in granulocytopenic patients. Intestinal IgA may be important, as deficient patients appear to be at an increased risk of infection. Transmission is primarily by the fecal-oral route, resulting in higher incidence in male homosexuals, retarded patients in institutions, and children in day-care centers.

347. APPLYING BASIC CONCEPTS: INITIAL WORKUP: ANSWER: B

348. APPLYING BASIC CONCEPTS: INITIAL WORKUP: ANSWER: C

(*Isselbacher, 13/e, p 1338.*) The central "scar" often seen in oncocytomas contains the central vessels that radiate out to the tumor's periphery in a spoke-wheel pattern. Lymphoma can involve the kidneys in several ways, but diffuse infiltration with smooth bilaterally enlarged kidneys is suggestive of lymphoma in the appropriate setting.

349. CLINICAL THERAPEUTICS: CONTINUED CARE: ANSWER: C

350. CLINICAL THERAPEUTICS: CONTINUED CARE: ANSWER: A

(Hardy, 2/e, pp 250-255.) Enflurane is a halogenated inhalation anesthetic with an MAC of 1.2. It is similar to halothane in its anesthetic characteristics. However, in a small number of normal patients it may induce electroencephalographic changes similar to those seen in epilepsy. Methoxyflurane is the most potent and least volatile halogenated inhalation anesthetic with an MAC of 0.16. Its clinical use has been curtailed because of the high risk of nephrotoxicity of the free fluoride ions released during its biodegradation. Morphine is a potent narcotic agent. Its use during general anesthesia can potentiate the analgesic effects of the inhalation agents. It causes histamine release with the risk of hypotension if given in a large bolus dose.

351. APPLYING BASIC CONCEPTS: CONTINUED CARE: ANSWER: C

352. APPLYING BASIC CONCEPTS: CONTINUED CARE: ANSWER: E

(*Isselbacher, 13/e, chap 81.*) Several distinct infectious syndromes have been linked to specific deficits in host defenses. Complement appears to be critical in the defense against neisserial infections since patients with deficiencies in the late components have recurrent *N. gonorrhoeae* and *meningitidis* infections. The spleen is one of the most important sites for phagocytosis of opsonized organisms. After splenectomy, whether surgical or functional as in sickle cell diseases, patients are at risk for development of bacteremia with organisms for which antibody forms the major host defense, such as *S. pneumoniae* and *Haemophilus influenzae.*

353. CLINICAL INTERVENTION: CONTINUED CARE: ANSWER: D

354. CLINICAL INTERVENTION: CONTINUED CARE: ANSWER: C

(Schwartz, 6/e, p 65.) One of the commonest causes of dehydration and metabolic disarray in surgical patients is the failure to replace gastrointestinal losses. External losses can often be collected for measurement of volume and ionic composition. Accurate replacement of these measured losses is clearly the best method of avoiding imbalance. However, a knowledge of the ionic composition of the intestinal contents at various sites permits an accurate estimate for early replacement. Most of these secretions start as extracellular fluid (with a composition similar to that of plasma) and are modified by intestinal glands. Colonic contents (stool) and saliva are most notable for their potassium content. The stomach substitutes hydrogen ions for sodium and thus eliminates all but a tiny fraction of bicarbonate.

355. CLINICAL THERAPEUTICS: CONTINUED CARE: ANSWER: D
356. CLINICAL THERAPEUTICS: CONTINUED CARE: ANSWER: D
357. CLINICAL THERAPEUTICS: CONTINUED CARE: ANSWER: A
(Isselbacher, 13/e, chap 367.) Rash and idiosyncratic bone marrow suppression are at times seen with phenobarbital, phenytoin, and carbamazepine; leukopenia and thrombocytopenia are most common with carbamazepine. Hepatotoxicity is a rare but feared effect of carbamazepine and an acute effect of valproic acid. In addition to the side effects listed in the question, phenytoin causes the appearance of a slightly prognathic jaw and coarsened facies. Phenytoin's neurologic side effects include ataxia. In fact, ataxia is a potential side effect of virtually all the anticonvulsants, including each of those listed in the question.

358. HISTORY AND PHYSICAL: CONTINUED CARE: ANSWER: D
359. HISTORY AND PHYSICAL: CONTINUED CARE: ANSWER: C
(Isselbacher, 13/e, chap 15.) In the assessment of uncomplicated disk protrusion, it is important to keep in mind that many lesions cause sciatica and that a protruding disk generally impinges on the nerve root that exits just below it (e.g., an "L5-S1 disk" most often compresses the Sl root). Walking on the toes requires a powerful gastrocnemius muscle, which is innervated by L5 and Sl. When weakness in this maneuver is coupled with a depressed ankle reflex, an Sl compression is likely (protrusion of the L5-Sl disk). Compression of the L5 root by an L4-L5 disk does not affect knee or ankle reflexes but causes anterior tibial weakness (foot-drop), extensor hallicus longus weakness, and weakness of foot inversion. The knee reflex is affected by an L3 or L4 radicular lesion (L2-L3 or L3-L4 disks, respectively), but hip flexors are affected by L2 and L3 only. These are the major lower extremity disk syndromes. In complex cases, several nerve roots are involved by protrusion of a single disk.

360. DIAGNOSIS: CONTINUED CARE: ANSWER: E
361. DIAGNOSIS: EMERGENCY: ANSWER: B
(*Eden, pp 749-766. Evans, pp 44-55, 60-71.*) A patient whose size is greater than her dates should always have an ultrasound examination to rule out multiple gestations.
Any bleeding during pregnancy should be investigated—especially heavy bleeding after the first trimester. The conditions that we are especially concerned about are placenta previa and low-lying placentas.

362. CLINICAL THERAPEUTICS: CONTINUED CARE: ANSWER: D
363. CLINICAL THERAPEUTICS: CONTINUED CARE: ANSWER: A
(*Isselbacher, 13/e, chap 318.*) Bleomycin is an antibiotic complex consisting of seven structurally related polypeptides. It both inhibits DNA synthesis and reacts with DNA to cause strand scission. Doxorubicin (Adriamycin), another antitumor antibiotic, inhibits DNA synthesis and DNA-dependent RNA synthesis. It acts by binding with DNA and causing untwisting of the helix which facilitates intercalation.

364. CLINICAL THERAPEUTICS: CONTINUED CARE: ANSWER: C
365. CLINICAL INTERVENTION: CONTINUED CARE: ANSWER: B
(*Isselbacher, 13/e, pp 1361-1362*) The nodular plaques seen in *Candida* esophagitis are due to the yeast itself and adjacent inflammation. *Herpes simplex* virus induces superficial erosions and associated vesicular lesion in the esophagus. Both *Herpes simplex* virus and *Candida* esophagitis typically occur in immunocompromised patients. Radiation esophagitis can occur following mediastinal radiation and can be potentiated by chemotherapeutic agents including bleomycin, doxorubicin, and cyclophosphamide. Doxycycline, tetracycline, and clindamycin are frequent causes of pill-induced esophagitis. Potassium chloride, aspirin, and ferrous sulphate are also common medications that are associated with this form of erosive esophagitis.

366. CLINICAL INTERVENTION: CONTINUED CARE: ANSWER: C
367. CLINICAL INTERVENTION: CONTINUED CARE: ANSWER: B
368. CLINICAL INTERVENTION: CONTINUED CARE: ANSWER: D
(*Evans, pp 136-140. Herbst, 2/e, pp 162, 449-453.*) Bleeding occurs in about 30 to 40 percent of human gestations before 20 weeks of pregnancy with about half of these pregnancies ending in spontaneous abortion. A threatened abortion takes place when this uterine bleeding occurs without any cervical dilation or effacement. In a patient bleeding during the first half of pregnancy, the diagnosis of inevitable abortion is strengthened if the bleeding is profuse and associated with uterine cramping pains. If cervical dilation has occurred, with or without rupture of membranes, the abortion is inevitable. If only a portion of the products of conception has been expelled and the cervix remains dilated, a diagnosis of incomplete abortion is made. However, if all fetal and placental tissue has been expelled, the cervix is closed, bleeding from the canal is minimal or decreasing, and uterine cramps have ceased, a diagnosis of complete abortion can be made. The diagnosis of missed abortion is suspected when the uterus fails to continue to enlarge with or without uterine bleeding or spotting. A missed abortion is one in which fetal death occurs before 20 weeks' gestation without expulsion of any fetal or maternal tissue for at least 8 weeks thereafter. When a fetus is retained in the uterus beyond 5 weeks after fetal death, consumptive coagulability with hypofibrogenemia may occur. This is uncommon, however, in gestations of less than 14 weeks' duration.

369. APPLYING BASIC CONCEPTS: INITIAL WORKUP: ANSWER: A
370. APPLYING BASIC CONCEPTS: INITIAL WORKUP: ANSWER: D
(*Isselbacher, 13/e, TABLE 257-2, p 1425.*)

371. DIAGNOSTIC STUDIES: INITIAL WORKUP: ANSWER: E
372. DIAGNOSTIC STUDIES: INITIAL WORKUP: ANSWER: A
(*Isselbacher, 13/e, chaps 201, 204, 206.*) Right heart failure, or elevated right-heart filling pressure, can develop from many causes. Right heart failure most commonly occurs as a result of pulmonary artery hypertension. Pulmonary artery hypertension, in turn, arises either from increased pulmonary vascular resistance with lung disease, in which case the pulmonary capillary wedge pressure (left atrial pressure) is not elevated, or from left-sided failure or valvular disease, in which case left atrial pressure is increased. Massive right ventricular infarction can cause the right side of the heart to fail at low systolic pressures. With primary myocardial disease, both left and right atrial pressures are elevated; however, when diastolic pressures are equal in the left and right cardiac chambers, external compression, such as constrictive pericarditis, must be suspected as the cause.

373. DIAGNOSTIC STUDIES: CONTINUED CARE: ANSWER: A
374. DIAGNOSTIC STUDIES: INITIAL WORKUP: ANSWER: B

(*Isselbacher, 13/e, pp 1495-1496.*) Cavernous hemangioma is a common benign lesion of the liver characterized by endothelial-lined vascular spaces. These spaces will accumulate labeled RBCs and can be definitively diagnosed with nuclear imaging. Frequently, however, the diagnosis is suspected based on ultrasound or CT findings and no further diagnostic workup is needed. Focal nodular hyperplasia is a benign liver mass that is unique among solid tumors of the liver in that it contains functioning Kupffer cells that will accumulate sulfur colloid. Thus, this lesion commonly will be "hot" or "warm" on sulfur colloid nuclear studies. Bile peritonitis may result from bile duct injury or inadequate cystic duct ligation which results in a communication between the biliary tree and the peritoneal space. The iminoacetic acid agents, the IDA family, will be taken up by the liver and excreted in the bile. Thus, these agents are useful in the detection of bile leaks. Because of the lipid soluability of xenon gas, there is increased deposition of this agent in the fatty liver. This is normally detected as an incidental finding on ventilation scintigrams as xenon gas is the agent often used in pulmonary ventilation studies.

375. DIAGNOSTIC STUDIES: INITIAL WORKUP: ANSWER: D
376. DIAGNOSTIC STUDIES: INITIAL WORKUP: ANSWER: B

(Schwartz, 6/e, pp 103-108.) The bleeding time assesses the interaction of platelets and the formation of the platelet plug. Therefore it will pick up deficiencies in both qualitative and quantitative platelet function. Ingestion of aspirin within 1 week of the test will alter the result.

The thrombin time assesses qualitative abnormalities in fibrinogen and the presence of inhibitors to fibrin polymerization. A standard amount of fibrin is added to a fixed volume of plasma and clotting time is measured.

Prothrombin time measures the speed of coagulation in the extrinsic pathway. A tissue source of procoagulant (thromboplastin) with calcium is added to plasma. The test will detect deficiencies in factors II, V, VII, X, and fibrinogen and is used to monitor patients receiving coumarin derivatives. However, even small amounts of heparin will artificially prolong the clotting time so that accurate prothrombin times can only be obtained when the patient has not received heparin for at least 5 h.

The intrinsic pathway is measured by the partial thromboplastin time. This test is sensitive for defects in factors VIII, IX, XI, XII, and all the factors of the extrinsic pathway and is used to monitor the status of patients on heparin.

377. HISTORY AND PHYSICAL: INITIAL WORKUP: ANSWER: E
378. APPLYING BASIC CONCEPTS: INITIAL WORKUP: ANSWER: C

(*Isselbacher, 13/e, TABLE 274-6, p 1531.*)

379. HEALTH MAINTENANCE: CONTINUED CARE: ANSWER: C
380. HEALTH MAINTENANCE: CONTINUED CARE: ANSWER: B
(*Evans, pp 111-116.*) Viral infections during pregnancy are of great concern. The risk to the fetus is greatest during the first trimester. Congenital infection in most instances results from transplacental transmission of the virus during maternal viremia. In addition, perinatal infection may result from acquisition of virus by passage of the infant through a contaminated birth canal. Cytomegalovirus, rubella, and varicella are well established as teratogens. Congenital disease may range from mild symptoms to major congenital defects to asymptomatic disease with late sequelae. Hepatitis B is only rarely transmitted in utero, but usually at the time of birth, and may cause a mild to severe hepatitis in infancy or, more commonly, result in a carrier state. Carriers run the risk of developing cirrhosis or hepatocellular carcinoma later in life. Rubeola is uncommon in pregnancy and has not been associated with any specific anomalies.

381. HEALTH MAINTENANCE: CONTINUED CARE: ANSWER: B
382. HEALTH MAINTENANCE: CONTINUED CARE: ANSWER: A
(*Isselbacher, 13/e, pp 1819, 2339.*) Certain hereditary conditions predispose to the development of neoplasia. The neurocutaneous disorders (Choices A, C, and D) are well known for this. Neurofibromatosis is highly associated with benign and malignant neural tumors as well as glial tumors and meningiomas. von Hippel-Lindau disease is associated with cerebellar hemangioblastomas, retinal angiomas, and renal cell carcinoma. Both disorders also have an association with pheochromocytomas. Tuberous sclerosis is characterized by glial tumors as well as renal angiomyofibromas and cardiac rhabdomyomas. Ataxia-telangiectasia is associated with lymphomas and leukemias. The increased incidence of malignancy in this disorder is felt to be due to chromosomal fragility.

383. HISTORY AND PHYSICAL: EMERGENCY: ANSWER: B
384. HISTORY AND PHYSICAL: CONTINUED CARE: ANSWER: A
(*Isselbacher, 13/e, chap 192.*) Equalization of diastolic pressures in the four cardiac chambers occurs in pericardial tamponade and constrictive pericarditis. The dip-and-plateau pattern in the ventricles and steep descent in the atria are features of constrictive pericarditis but not pericardial tamponade. In persons who have restrictive cardiomyopathy, diastolic pressures may be nearly equal. Often, however, a separation of at least 5 mmHg exists or can be brought out by acute volume loading. The dip-and-plateau pattern in ventricular pressures is typical.

385. HEALTH MAINTENANCE: EMERGENCY: ANSWER: D
386. PROGNOSIS: EMERGENCY: ANSWER: C
(*Schwartz, 6/e, pp 1900-1934.*) Fractures of the navicular bone of the wrist should be suspected in anyone, particularly a young person, who falls on an outstretched hand. Although x-rays are mandatory, it is important to realize that the fracture may not be seen on the initial x-ray and that a presumptive diagnosis can and should be made on clinical grounds alone. Typically, there will be tenderness to palpation over the navicular tuberosity and limitation of wrist flexion and extension. Immobilization of the wrist for about 16 weeks and sometimes up to 6 months is required. Nonunion or avascular necrosis is not uncommon and may require bone grafting for correction. Anterior shoulder dislocations occur more frequently than posterior dislocations. However, posterior dislocations are seen in special situations, such as during an epileptiform convulsion and during electroshock therapy. Closed reduction followed by immobilization is usually sufficient therapy.

387. HISTORY AND PHYSICAL: CONTINUED CARE: ANSWER: D
388. HISTORY AND PHYSICAL: CONTINUED CARE: ANSWER: A
(Isselbacher, 13/e, chaps 199, 222.) Many hereditary conditions and exposures to infectious agents during pregnancy result in congenital heart disease. Marfan's syndrome is a disorder of connective tissue in which cardiac abnormalities produce the greatest mortality. Decreased strength of the aortic connective tissue results in dilatation with aortic regurgitation and aortic dissection. Prolapse of the aortic and mitral valves usually presents, the latter associated with mitral regurgitation. Turner's syndrome is a chromosomal abnormality (45, XO) characterized by short stature and hypogonadism. Associated cardiac defects include coarctation of the aorta and bicuspid aortic valve.

389. HISTORY AND PHYSICAL: INITIAL WORKUP: ANSWER: C
390. HEALTH MAINTENANCE: CONTINUED CARE: ANSWER: B
(*Ryan, 5/e, pp 117-121, 591-595.*) Many cases of nonspecific vaginitis are caused by *Gardnerella vaginalis.* Women with this infection usually complain of a characteristically malodorous, grayish vaginal discharge. On wet mounts, the diagnosis is made by visualizing the "clue cells," which are epithelial cells with large numbers of adherent coccobacilli. The recommended treatment is ampicillin, although vaginal sulfa creams are also effective. Besides diabetes mellitus, other predisposing factors of candidiasis include pregnancy, the use of antibiotics, immunosuppressive medications, and possibly oral contraceptives. Affected women usually complain of severe pruritus and a thick, cheeselike vaginal discharge. Wet mounts show characteristic yeast cells and hyphae. The primary mode of treatment is the vaginal application of an antifungal agent, such as nystatin.
Trichomonas vaginalis classically gives rise to a yellowish, frothy discharge, which is foul-smelling and causes pruritus.

391. DIAGNOSTIC STUDIES: CONTINUED CARE: ANSWER: C
392. DIAGNOSTIC STUDIES: CONTINUED CARE: ANSWER: B
(*Isselbacher, 13/e, TABLE 307-2, p 1744.*)

393. DIAGNOSTIC STUDIES: CONTINUED CARE: ANSWER: A
394. DIAGNOSTIC STUDIES: CONTINUED CARE: ANSWER: B
(Silverman, 8/e, pp 1629, 1633.) Infantile polycystic kidney disease is an autosomal recessive condition in which infants present with symmetrically enlarged kidneys that are echogenic due to the myriad tissue interfaces presented by the dilated tubules and collecting ducts. Oliguria and secondary pulmonary hypoplasia may occur in utero, leading to respiratory distress shortly after birth.
Communicating cystic structures, representing the dilated renal collecting system, are the ultrasound hallmark of hydronephrosis. In contrast, the multicystic dysplastic kidney consists of noncommunicating cysts of varying sizes separated by varying amounts of dysplastic parenchyma. The ureter is often atretic in the region of the ureteropelvic junction.

395. DIAGNOSTIC STUDIES: CONTINUED CARE: ANSWER: C
396. DIAGNOSTIC STUDIES: CONTINUED CARE: ANSWER: A
(*Isselbacher, 13/e, pp 325, 1621, 1773, 1777.*) The cytoplasmic extensions noted occasionally on smear and consistently with phase microscopy give a "hairy" appearance to these cells. The Reed-Sternberg cell can be seen in non-Hodgkin's lymphomas rarely but is the hallmark of Hodgkin's disease. The lytic defects and osteoporosis seen with myeloma are due to the osteoclast-activating factor produced by the myeloma cells. Diseases associated with a proliferation of either tissue macrophages (histiocytes) or special bone marrow-derived cells called Langerhan's cells are termed histiocytoses.

397. DIAGNOSIS: INITIAL WORKUP: ANSWER: A
398. DIAGNOSIS: INITIAL WORKUP: ANSWER: C
(Taveras & Ferrucci, vol 2, chap 94 and 109. Gedgaudas, chaps 5-9.) When presented with a case in which congenital heart disease may be present, it is often helpful to focus the differential possibilities by addressing the presence or absence of cyanosis and the condition of the pulmonary vascularity.
Cyanosis with increased pulmonary blood flow is typical of the admixture lesions, in which deoxygenated blood is allowed to enter the systemic circulation. Typically, the shunt is bidirectional, and the pulmonic circulation receives greater-than-normal flow. The most common of these are the "T" lesions described by Elliott: transposition of the great vessels, truncus arteriosus, and total anomalous pulmonary venous return. In the latter, one-fourth of patients have obstruction of the abnormal vein, producing pulmonary venous congestion. However, many nonobstructed patients will develop congestive heart failure due to the increased demand on the right ventricle.
The condition of increased pulmonary blood flow, in the absence of cyanosis, indicates a left-to-right shunt. Most common are ventricular septal defect (VSD), atrial septal defect (ASD), and patent ductus arteriosus (PDA). To help differentiate these, determination of the left atrial size is the next step. If it is enlarged, then ASD and endocardial cushion defect can be excluded because the extra blood volume flows immediately into the lower-pressure right atrium. The next step is to evaluate the aorta. If the aortic knob is markedly diminished in size, this indicates that the shunt is intracardiac and a VSD is likely. An extracardiac shunt, such as a PDA, tends to equalize the size of the aorta and pulmonary artery.
Ebstein anomaly is one of several lesions which results in functional right ventricular (RV) outflow obstruction, and hence diminished pulmonary vascularity. These patients shunt right to left at the atrial level through a patent foramen ovale or ASD, producing cyanosis which is usually present shortly after birth. The most common cause of decreased pulmonary vascularity and cyanosis is tetralogy of Fallot. Tricuspid atresia, pulmonary stenosis, and Uhl anomaly (deficient RV myocardium) are other causes.

399. CLINICAL THERAPEUTICS: CONTINUED CARE: ANSWER: B
400. CLINICAL THERAPEUTICS: CONTINUED CARE: ANSWER: H
(*DiSaia, 4/e, pp 376-381.*) Cyclophosphamide is an alkylating agent that cross-links DNA and also inhibits DNA synthesis. Hemorrhagic cystitis and alopecia are common side effects. Cisplatin causes renal damage and neural toxicity. Patients must be well hydrated. Its mode of action does not fit a specific category.

Bibliography

Bibliography

Amplatz K, Moller J, Castañeda-Zuñiga W: *Radiology of Congenital Heart Disease.* Philadelphia, Thieme Medical, 1986.

Anderson RJ, et al: Unrecognized adult salicylate intoxication. *Ann Intern Med* 85:745-748, 1976.

Armstrong P, Wilson AG, Dee P: *Imaging of the Diseases of the Chest.* Chicago, Year Book Medical, 1990.

Balow JE, Austin HA, Tsokos GC, et al: Lupus nephritis. *Ann Intern Med* 106:79-94, 1987.

Barron WM, Lindheimer MD (eds): *Medical Disorders During Pregnancy.* St. Louis, Mosby, 1991.

Becker L, et al (eds): *Principles and Practice of Endocrinology and Metabolism.* Philadelphia, Lippincott, 1990.

Behrman RE: *Nelson Textbook of Pediatrics,* 14/e. Philadelphia, WB Saunders, 1992.

Behrman SJ, Kistner RW, Patten GW (eds): *Progress in Infertility,* 3/e. Boston, Little, Brown, 1988.

Berek JS, Hacker NF (eds): *Practical Gynecologic Oncology.* Baltimore, Williams & Wilkins, 1989.

Brooks J: *Surgery of the Pancreas.* Philadelphia, WB Saunders, 1983.

Burrow GN, Ferris TF: *Medical Complications during Pregnancy,* 3/e. Philadelphia, WB Saunders, 1988.

Byrne JJ, Moake JL: Thrombotic thrombocytopenic purpura and the hemolytic uremic syndrome: Evolving concepts of pathogenesis and therapy. *Baillieres Clin Haematol* 15:413-442, 1986.

Cameron JL: *Current Surgical Therapy,* 4/e. St. Louis, Mosby, 1992.

Carmichael KA, Fallon MD, Dalinka M, et al: Osteomalacia and osteitis fibrosa in a man ingesting aluminum hydroxide antacid. *Am J Med* 76: 1137-1143, 1984.

Carr BR, Blackwell RE (eds): *Textbook of Reproductive Medicine.* East Norwalk, CT, Appleton & Lange, 1993.

Charles D, et al (eds): *Handbook of Infectious Diseases: Obstetric and Perinatal Infections.* St. Louis, Mosby, 1993.

Cunningham FG, et al (eds): *Williams Obstetrics,* 19/e. East Norwalk, CT, Appleton & Lange, 1993.

Curran JW, Jaffe HW, Hardy AM, et al: Epidemiology of HIV infection and AIDS in the United States. *Science* 239:610-616, 1988.

Davis JH, et al (eds): *Clinical Surgery.* St. Louis, CV Mosby, 1987.

DiSaia PJ, Creasman WT (eds): *Clinical Gynecologic Oncology,* 4/e. St. Louis, Mosby, 1993.

Droegemueller W, et al (eds): *Comprehensive Gynecology.* St. Louis, CV Mosby, 1987.

Eden RD, Boehm FH (eds): *Assessment and Care of the Fetus: Physiological, Clinical, and Medicolegal Principles.* East Norwalk, CT, Appleton & Lange, 1990.

Evans MI (ed): *Reproductive Risks and Prenatal Diagnosis.* East Norwalk, CT, Appleton & Lange, 1992.

Fisher CM: Lacunar strokes and infarcts: A review. *Neurology* 32:871-876, 1982.

Gabuzda DH, Hirsch MS: Neurologic manifestations of infection with human immunodeficiency virus. Clinical features and pathogenesis. *Ann Intern Med* 107:383-391, 1987.

Gedgaudas E, Moller JH, Castañeda-Zuñiga WR, Amplatz K: *Cardiovascular Radiology.* Philadelphia, WB Saunders, 1985.

Gomel V, et al: Gynecology*: A Practical Approach.* Baltimore, Williams & Wilkins, 1990.

Greenberger PA, Patterson R: Allergic bronchopulmonary aspergillosis. Model of bronchopulmonary disease with defined serologic, radiologic, pathologic and clinical findings from asthma to fatal destructive lung diseases. *Chest* 91(S6):165S-171S, 1987.

Hardy JT (ed): *Hardy's Textbook of Surgery,* 2/e. Philadelphia, JB Lippincott, 1988.

Henderson ES, Lister TA (eds): *Leukemia,* 5/e. Philadelphia, WB Saunders, 1990.

Herbst AL, et al (eds): *Comprehensive Gynecology,* 2/e. St. Louis, Mosby, 1992.

Hochberg FH, Miller DC: Primary central nervous system lymphoma. *J Neurosurg* 68:835-853, 1988.

Isselbacher KJ, et al (eds): *Harrison's Principles of Internal Medicine,* 13/e. New York, McGraw-Hill, 1994.

Jandl JH: *Blood—A Textbook of Hematology.* Boston, Little, Brown, 1987.

Jones KL (ed): *Smith's Recognizable Patterns of Human Malformations,* 4/e. Philadelphia, Saunders, 1988.

Kase NG, et al: *Principles and Practice of Clinical Gynecology,* 2/e. New York, Churchill Livingstone, 1990.

Kelly WN, Harris ED Jr, Ruddy S, Sledge CB: *Textbook of Rheumatology.* Philadelphia, WB Saunders, 1989.

Kurman RJ (ed): *Blaustein's Pathology of the Female Genital Tract,* 4/e. New York, Springer-Verlag, 1994.

Lee GR: The anemia of chronic disease. *Semin Hematol* 20:61-80, 1983.

Malech HL, Gallin JI: Neutrophils in human diseases. *N Engl J Med* 317:687-694, 1987.

Mandell GL, et al: *Principles and Practice of Infectious Diseases,* 3/e. New York, Churchill Livingstone, 1990.

Martin JB, Gusella JF: Huntington's disease: Pathogenesis and management. *N Engl J Med* 315:1267-1276, 1986.

Mattingly RF, Thompson JD: *TeLinde's Operative Gynecology,* 6/e. Philadelphia, JB Lippincott, 1986.

Muller JE, Rude RE, Braunwald EB, et al: Myocardial infarct extension: Occurrence, outcome, and risk factors in the multicenter investigation of limitation of infarct size. *Ann Intern Med* 108:1-6, 1988.

Nichols DH (ed): *Gynecologic and Obstetric Surgery.* St. Louis, Mosby, 1993.

Pizzo PA, Commers J, Cotton D, et al: Approaching the controversies in antibacterial management of cancer patients. *Am J Med* 76:436-449, 1984.

Reece EA, et al (eds): *Medicine of the Fetus and Mother.* Philadelphia, Lippincott, 1992.

Remington JS, Klein JO (eds): *Infectious Diseases of the Fetus and Newborn Infant,* 3/e. Philadelphia, Saunders, 1992.

Rich S: Primary pulmonary hypertension. *Prog Cardiovasc Dis* 31:205-238, 1988.

Rosse WF, Parker CJ: Paroxysmal nocturnal hemoglobinuria. *Clin Haematol* 14:105-125, 1985.

Rudolph AM: *Rudolph Pediatrics,* 19/e. East Norwalk, CT, Appleton & Lange, 1991.

Ryan KJ, et al: *Kistner's Gynecology: Principles and Practice,* 5/e. Chicago, Year Book Medical, 1990.

Sabiston DC Jr: *Textbook of Surgery: The Biological Basis of Modern Surgical Practice,* 13/e. Philadelphia, WB Saunders, 1986.

Schwartz GF, et al: Significance and staging of nonpalpable carcinomas of the breast. *Surg Gynecol Obstet* 166:6-10, 1988.

Schwartz SI, Shires GT, Spencer FC (eds): *Principles of Surgery,* 6/e. New York, McGraw-Hill, 1993.

Shiau YF, Feldman GM, Resnick MA, et al: Stool electrolyte and osmolality measurements in the evaluation of diarrheal disorders. *Ann Intern Med* 102:773-775, 1985.

Shires GT (ed): *Principles of Trauma Care,* 3/e. New York, McGraw-Hill, 1985.

Silverman FN, Kuhn JP: *Essentials of Caffey's Pediatric X-Ray Diagnosis.* Chicago, Year Book Medical, 1990.

Speroff L, Glass R: *Clinical Gynecologic Endocrinology and Infertility,* 4/e. Baltimore, Williams & Wilkins, 1989.

Steere AC: Lyme disease. *N Engl J Med* 321:586-596, 1989.

Tandan R, Bradley WG: Amyotrophic lateral sclerosis: Part I. Clinical features, pathology, and ethical issues in management. *Ann Neurol* 18:271-280, 1985.

Taveras JM, Ferrucci JT (eds): *Radiology: Diagnosis Imaging-Intervention.* Philadelphia, JB Lippincott, 1990.

The TIMI Study Group: Comparison of invasive and conservative strategies after treatment with intravenous tissue plasminogen activator in acute myocardial infarction: Results of the thrombolysis in myocardial infarction (TIMI) phase II trial. *N Engl J Med* 320:618-627, 1989.

Trotman IF, Misiewicz JJ: Sigmoid motility in diverticular disease and the irritable bowel syndrome. *Gut* 29:218-222, 1988.

Verkauf BS (ed): *Congenital Malformations of the Female Reproductive Tract and Their Treatment.* East Norwalk, CT, Appleton & Lange, 1993.

Vogelstein B, Fearon ER, Hamilton SR, et al: Genetic alterations during colorectal-tumor development. *N Engl J Med* 319:525-532, 1988.

Walt AJ: *Early Care of the Injured Patient,* 3/e. Philadelphia, WB Saunders, 1982.

Wilmore DW, Brennan MF, Harken AH, et al (eds): *Care of the Surgical Patient.* New York, Scientific American Books, 1990.

Youmans JR (ed): *Neurological Surgery,* 3/e. Philadelphia, WB Saunders, 1990.

Young GA, Vincent PC: Drug-induced agranulocytosis. *Clin Haematol* 9:483-504, 1980.

Index

D

E

F

G

H

I

R

S

T

Answer Sheets

ANSWER SHEET FOR BOOK A

001 [A] [B] [C] [D] [E]
002 [A] [B] [C] [D] [E]
003 [A] [B] [C] [D] [E]
004 [A] [B] [C] [D] [E]
005 [A] [B] [C] [D] [E]
006 [A] [B] [C] [D] [E]
007 [A] [B] [C] [D] [E]
008 [A] [B] [C] [D] [E]
009 [A] [B] [C] [D] [E]
010 [A] [B] [C] [D] [E]
011 [A] [B] [C] [D] [E]
012 [A] [B] [C] [D] [E]
013 [A] [B] [C] [D] [E]
014 [A] [B] [C] [D] [E]
015 [A] [B] [C] [D] [E]
016 [A] [B] [C] [D] [E]
017 [A] [B] [C] [D] [E]
018 [A] [B] [C] [D] [E]
019 [A] [B] [C] [D] [E]
020 [A] [B] [C] [D] [E]
021 [A] [B] [C] [D] [E]
022 [A] [B] [C] [D] [E]
023 [A] [B] [C] [D] [E]
024 [A] [B] [C] [D] [E]
025 [A] [B] [C] [D] [E]
026 [A] [B] [C] [D] [E]
027 [A] [B] [C] [D] [E]
028 [A] [B] [C] [D] [E]
029 [A] [B] [C] [D] [E]
030 [A] [B] [C] [D] [E]
031 [A] [B] [C] [D] [E]
032 [A] [B] [C] [D] [E]
033 [A] [B] [C] [D] [E]
034 [A] [B] [C] [D] [E]
035 [A] [B] [C] [D] [E]
036 [A] [B] [C] [D] [E]
037 [A] [B] [C] [D] [E]
038 [A] [B] [C] [D] [E]
039 [A] [B] [C] [D] [E]
040 [A] [B] [C] [D] [E]
041 [A] [B] [C] [D] [E]
042 [A] [B] [C] [D] [E]
043 [A] [B] [C] [D] [E]
044 [A] [B] [C] [D] [E]
045 [A] [B] [C] [D] [E]
046 [A] [B] [C] [D] [E]
047 [A] [B] [C] [D] [E]
048 [A] [B] [C] [D] [E]
049 [A] [B] [C] [D] [E]
050 [A] [B] [C] [D] [E]
051 [A] [B] [C] [D] [E]
052 [A] [B] [C] [D] [E]
053 [A] [B] [C] [D] [E]
054 [A] [B] [C] [D] [E]
055 [A] [B] [C] [D] [E]
056 [A] [B] [C] [D] [E]
057 [A] [B] [C] [D] [E]
058 [A] [B] [C] [D] [E]
059 [A] [B] [C] [D] [E]
060 [A] [B] [C] [D] [E]
061 [A] [B] [C] [D] [E]
062 [A] [B] [C] [D] [E]
063 [A] [B] [C] [D] [E]
064 [A] [B] [C] [D] [E]
065 [A] [B] [C] [D] [E]
066 [A] [B] [C] [D] [E]
067 [A] [B] [C] [D] [E]
068 [A] [B] [C] [D] [E]
069 [A] [B] [C] [D] [E]
070 [A] [B] [C] [D] [E]
071 [A] [B] [C] [D] [E]
072 [A] [B] [C] [D] [E]
073 [A] [B] [C] [D] [E]
074 [A] [B] [C] [D] [E]
075 [A] [B] [C] [D] [E]
076 [A] [B] [C] [D] [E]
077 [A] [B] [C] [D] [E]
078 [A] [B] [C] [D] [E]
079 [A] [B] [C] [D] [E]
080 [A] [B] [C] [D] [E]
081 [A] [B] [C] [D] [E]
082 [A] [B] [C] [D] [E]
083 [A] [B] [C] [D] [E]
084 [A] [B] [C] [D] [E]
085 [A] [B] [C] [D] [E]
086 [A] [B] [C] [D] [E]
087 [A] [B] [C] [D] [E]
088 [A] [B] [C] [D] [E]
089 [A] [B] [C] [D] [E]
090 [A] [B] [C] [D] [E]
091 [A] [B] [C] [D] [E]
092 [A] [B] [C] [D] [E]
093 [A] [B] [C] [D] [E]
094 [A] [B] [C] [D] [E]
095 [A] [B] [C] [D] [E]
096 [A] [B] [C] [D] [E]
097 [A] [B] [C] [D] [E]
098 [A] [B] [C] [D] [E]
099 [A] [B] [C] [D] [E]
100 [A] [B] [C] [D] [E]
101 [A] [B] [C] [D] [E]
102 [A] [B] [C] [D] [E]

103 [A] [B] [C] [D] [E]

104 [A] [B] [C] [D] [E]

105 [A] [B] [C] [D] [E]

106 [A] [B] [C] [D] [E]

107 [A] [B] [C] [D] [E]

108 [A] [B] [C] [D] [E]

109 [A] [B] [C] [D] [E]

110 [A] [B] [C] [D] [E]

111 [A] [B] [C] [D] [E]

112 [A] [B] [C] [D] [E]

113 [A] [B] [C] [D] [E]

114 [A] [B] [C] [D] [E]

115 [A] [B] [C] [D] [E]

116 [A] [B] [C] [D] [E]

117 [A] [B] [C] [D] [E]

118 [A] [B] [C] [D] [E]

119 [A] [B] [C] [D] [E]

120 [A] [B] [C] [D] [E]

121 [A] [B] [C] [D] [E]

122 [A] [B] [C] [D] [E]

123 [A] [B] [C] [D] [E]

124 [A] [B] [C] [D] [E]

125 [A] [B] [C] [D] [E]

126 [A] [B] [C] [D] [E]

127 [A] [B] [C] [D] [E]

128 [A] [B] [C] [D] [E]

129 [A] [B] [C] [D] [E]

130 [A] [B] [C] [D] [E]

131 [A] [B] [C] [D] [E]

132 [A] [B] [C] [D] [E]

133 [A] [B] [C] [D] [E]

134 [A] [B] [C] [D] [E]

135 [A] [B] [C] [D] [E]

136 [A] [B] [C] [D] [E]

137 [A] [B] [C] [D] [E]

138 [A] [B] [C] [D] [E]

139 [A] [B] [C] [D] [E]

140 [A] [B] [C] [D] [E]

141 [A] [B] [C] [D] [E]

142 [A] [B] [C] [D] [E]

143 [A] [B] [C] [D] [E]

144 [A] [B] [C] [D] [E]

145 [A] [B] [C] [D] [E]

146 [A] [B] [C] [D] [E]

147 [A] [B] [C] [D] [E]

148 [A] [B] [C] [D] [E]

149 [A] [B] [C] [D] [E]

150 [A] [B] [C] [D] [E]

151 [A] [B] [C] [D] [E]

152 [A] [B] [C] [D] [E]

153 [A] [B] [C] [D] [E]

154 [A] [B] [C] [D] [E]

155 [A] [B] [C] [D] [E]

156 [A] [B] [C] [D] [E]

157 [A] [B] [C] [D] [E]

158 [A] [B] [C] [D] [E]

159 [A] [B] [C] [D] [E]

160 [A] [B] [C] [D] [E]

161 [A] [B] [C] [D] [E]

162 [A] [B] [C] [D] [E]

163 [A] [B] [C] [D] [E]

164 [A] [B] [C] [D] [E]

165 [A] [B] [C] [D] [E]

166 [A] [B] [C] [D] [E]

167 [A] [B] [C] [D] [E]

168 [A] [B] [C] [D] [E]

169 [A] [B] [C] [D] [E]

170 [A] [B] [C] [D] [E]

171 [A] [B] [C] [D] [E]

172 [A] [B] [C] [D] [E]

173 [A] [B] [C] [D] [E]

174 [A] [B] [C] [D] [E]

175 [A] [B] [C] [D] [E]

176 [A] [B] [C] [D] [E]

177 [A] [B] [C] [D] [E]

178 [A] [B] [C] [D] [E]

179 [A] [B] [C] [D] [E]

180 [A] [B] [C] [D] [E]

181 [A] [B] [C] [D] [E]

182 [A] [B] [C] [D] [E]

183 [A] [B] [C] [D] [E]

184 [A] [B] [C] [D] [E]

185 [A] [B] [C] [D] [E]

186 [A] [B] [C] [D] [E]

187 [A] [B] [C] [D] [E]

188 [A] [B] [C] [D] [E]

189 [A] [B] [C] [D] [E]

190 [A] [B] [C] [D] [E]

191 [A] [B] [C] [D] [E]

192 [A] [B] [C] [D] [E]

193 [A] [B] [C] [D] [E]
[F] [G] [H] [I] [J]

194 [A] [B] [C] [D] [E]
[F] [G] [H] [I] [J]

195 [A] [B] [C] [D] [E]
[F] [G] [H] [I] [J]

196 [A] [B] [C] [D] [E]
[F] [G] [H] [I] [J]

197 [A] [B] [C] [D] [E]
[F] [G] [H] [I] [J]

198 [A] [B] [C] [D] [E]
[F] [G] [H] [I] [J]

199 [A] [B] [C] [D] [E]
[F] [G] [H] [I] [J]

200 [A] [B] [C] [D] [E]
[F] [G] [H] [I] [J]

ANSWER SHEET FOR BOOK B

201 [A] [B] [C] [D] [E]
202 [A] [B] [C] [D] [E]
203 [A] [B] [C] [D] [E]
204 [A] [B] [C] [D] [E]
205 [A] [B] [C] [D] [E]
206 [A] [B] [C] [D] [E]
207 [A] [B] [C] [D] [E]
208 [A] [B] [C] [D] [E]
209 [A] [B] [C] [D] [E]
210 [A] [B] [C] [D] [E]
211 [A] [B] [C] [D] [E]
212 [A] [B] [C] [D] [E]
213 [A] [B] [C] [D] [E]
214 [A] [B] [C] [D] [E]
215 [A] [B] [C] [D] [E]
216 [A] [B] [C] [D] [E]
217 [A] [B] [C] [D] [E]
218 [A] [B] [C] [D] [E]
219 [A] [B] [C] [D] [E]
220 [A] [B] [C] [D] [E]
221 [A] [B] [C] [D] [E]
222 [A] [B] [C] [D] [E]
223 [A] [B] [C] [D] [E]
224 [A] [B] [C] [D] [E]
225 [A] [B] [C] [D] [E]
226 [A] [B] [C] [D] [E]
227 [A] [B] [C] [D] [E]
228 [A] [B] [C] [D] [E]
229 [A] [B] [C] [D] [E]
230 [A] [B] [C] [D] [E]
231 [A] [B] [C] [D] [E]
232 [A] [B] [C] [D] [E]
233 [A] [B] [C] [D] [E]
234 [A] [B] [C] [D] [E]
235 [A] [B] [C] [D] [E]
236 [A] [B] [C] [D] [E]
237 [A] [B] [C] [D] [E]
238 [A] [B] [C] [D] [E]
239 [A] [B] [C] [D] [E]
240 [A] [B] [C] [D] [E]
241 [A] [B] [C] [D] [E]
242 [A] [B] [C] [D] [E]
243 [A] [B] [C] [D] [E]
244 [A] [B] [C] [D] [E]
245 [A] [B] [C] [D] [E]
246 [A] [B] [C] [D] [E]
247 [A] [B] [C] [D] [E]
248 [A] [B] [C] [D] [E]
249 [A] [B] [C] [D] [E]
250 [A] [B] [C] [D] [E]
251 [A] [B] [C] [D] [E]
252 [A] [B] [C] [D] [E]
253 [A] [B] [C] [D] [E]
254 [A] [B] [C] [D] [E]
255 [A] [B] [C] [D] [E]
256 [A] [B] [C] [D] [E]
257 [A] [B] [C] [D] [E]
258 [A] [B] [C] [D] [E]
259 [A] [B] [C] [D] [E]
260 [A] [B] [C] [D] [E]
261 [A] [B] [C] [D] [E]
262 [A] [B] [C] [D] [E]
263 [A] [B] [C] [D] [E]
264 [A] [B] [C] [D] [E]
265 [A] [B] [C] [D] [E]
266 [A] [B] [C] [D] [E]
267 [A] [B] [C] [D] [E]
268 [A] [B] [C] [D] [E]
269 [A] [B] [C] [D] [E]
270 [A] [B] [C] [D] [E]
271 [A] [B] [C] [D] [E]
272 [A] [B] [C] [D] [E]
273 [A] [B] [C] [D] [E]
274 [A] [B] [C] [D] [E]
275 [A] [B] [C] [D] [E]
276 [A] [B] [C] [D] [E]
277 [A] [B] [C] [D] [E]
278 [A] [B] [C] [D] [E]
279 [A] [B] [C] [D] [E]
280 [A] [B] [C] [D] [E]
281 [A] [B] [C] [D] [E]
282 [A] [B] [C] [D] [E]
283 [A] [B] [C] [D] [E]
284 [A] [B] [C] [D] [E]
285 [A] [B] [C] [D] [E]
286 [A] [B] [C] [D] [E]
287 [A] [B] [C] [D] [E]
288 [A] [B] [C] [D] [E]
289 [A] [B] [C] [D] [E]
290 [A] [B] [C] [D] [E]
291 [A] [B] [C] [D] [E]
292 [A] [B] [C] [D] [E]
293 [A] [B] [C] [D] [E]
294 [A] [B] [C] [D] [E]
295 [A] [B] [C] [D] [E]
296 [A] [B] [C] [D] [E]
297 [A] [B] [C] [D] [E]
298 [A] [B] [C] [D] [E]
299 [A] [B] [C] [D] [E]
300 [A] [B] [C] [D] [E]
301 [A] [B] [C] [D] [E]
302 [A] [B] [C] [D] [E]

303 [A] [B] [C] [D] [E]
304 [A] [B] [C] [D] [E]
305 [A] [B] [C] [D] [E]
306 [A] [B] [C] [D] [E]
307 [A] [B] [C] [D] [E]
308 [A] [B] [C] [D] [E]
309 [A] [B] [C] [D] [E]
310 [A] [B] [C] [D] [E]
311 [A] [B] [C] [D] [E]
312 [A] [B] [C] [D] [E]
313 [A] [B] [C] [D] [E]
314 [A] [B] [C] [D] [E]
315 [A] [B] [C] [D] [E]
316 [A] [B] [C] [D] [E]
317 [A] [B] [C] [D] [E]
318 [A] [B] [C] [D] [E]
319 [A] [B] [C] [D] [E]
320 [A] [B] [C] [D] [E]
321 [A] [B] [C] [D] [E]
322 [A] [B] [C] [D] [E]
323 [A] [B] [C] [D] [E]
324 [A] [B] [C] [D] [E]
325 [A] [B] [C] [D] [E]
326 [A] [B] [C] [D] [E]
327 [A] [B] [C] [D] [E]
328 [A] [B] [C] [D] [E]
329 [A] [B] [C] [D] [E]
330 [A] [B] [C] [D] [E]
331 [A] [B] [C] [D] [E]
332 [A] [B] [C] [D] [E]
333 [A] [B] [C] [D] [E]
334 [A] [B] [C] [D] [E]
335 [A] [B] [C] [D] [E]
336 [A] [B] [C] [D] [E]
337 [A] [B] [C] [D] [E]
338 [A] [B] [C] [D] [E]
339 [A] [B] [C] [D] [E]
340 [A] [B] [C] [D] [E]
341 [A] [B] [C] [D] [E]
342 [A] [B] [C] [D] [E]
343 [A] [B] [C] [D] [E]
344 [A] [B] [C] [D] [E]
345 [A] [B] [C] [D] [E]
346 [A] [B] [C] [D] [E]
347 [A] [B] [C] [D] [E]
348 [A] [B] [C] [D] [E]
349 [A] [B] [C] [D] [E]
350 [A] [B] [C] [D] [E]
351 [A] [B] [C] [D] [E]
352 [A] [B] [C] [D] [E]
353 [A] [B] [C] [D] [E]
354 [A] [B] [C] [D] [E]
355 [A] [B] [C] [D] [E]
356 [A] [B] [C] [D] [E]
357 [A] [B] [C] [D] [E]
358 [A] [B] [C] [D] [E]
359 [A] [B] [C] [D] [E]
360 [A] [B] [C] [D] [E]
361 [A] [B] [C] [D] [E]
362 [A] [B] [C] [D] [E]
363 [A] [B] [C] [D] [E]
364 [A] [B] [C] [D] [E]
365 [A] [B] [C] [D] [E]
366 [A] [B] [C] [D] [E]
367 [A] [B] [C] [D] [E]
368 [A] [B] [C] [D] [E]
369 [A] [B] [C] [D] [E]
370 [A] [B] [C] [D] [E]
371 [A] [B] [C] [D] [E]
372 [A] [B] [C] [D] [E]
373 [A] [B] [C] [D] [E]
374 [A] [B] [C] [D] [E]
375 [A] [B] [C] [D] [E]
376 [A] [B] [C] [D] [E]
377 [A] [B] [C] [D] [E]
378 [A] [B] [C] [D] [E]
379 [A] [B] [C] [D] [E]
380 [A] [B] [C] [D] [E]
381 [A] [B] [C] [D] [E]
382 [A] [B] [C] [D] [E]
383 [A] [B] [C] [D] [E]
384 [A] [B] [C] [D] [E]
385 [A] [B] [C] [D] [E]
386 [A] [B] [C] [D] [E]
387 [A] [B] [C] [D] [E]
388 [A] [B] [C] [D] [E]
389 [A] [B] [C] [D] [E]
390 [A] [B] [C] [D] [E]
391 [A] [B] [C] [D] [E]
392 [A] [B] [C] [D] [E]
393 [A] [B] [C] [D] [E]
394 [A] [B] [C] [D] [E]
395 [A] [B] [C] [D] [E]
396 [A] [B] [C] [D] [E]
397 [A] [B] [C] [D] [E]
398 [A] [B] [C] [D] [E]
399 [A] [B] [C] [D] [E]
[F] [G] [H] [I] [J]
400 [A] [B] [C] [D] [E]
[F] [G] [H] [I] [J]